THE
SPIRIT
OF
EXCELLENCE

How Health Care Organizations Are Achieving Service, Quality & Satisfaction

Edited by
KRISTINE PETERSON

CANDENT PRESS
Chicago, Illinois

Cover Design: Terry Ernsberger

First Edition

ISBN: 0-9760461-0-5

The content of this book was submitted by health care organizations, and it is the hospitals and residential care facilities featured in this book that I appreciate most of all. Thank you for your willingness to be included.

I would like to thank those who have authored entries to the Sodexho Spirit of Excellence award program over the previous 12 years and acknowledge the thousands of individuals who have contributed to the successes these entries represent. I have benefited professionally by what I have learned from your initiatives, and as a consumer, I am and will remain indebted to you for your continuous efforts to improve my health and aging experiences.

In 1992, Clark Bell, as editor of *Modern Healthcare*, invited me to judge the first award competition. For the opportunities he introduced and continued to extend, I am very appreciative.

I have known Chuck Lauer for more than 20 years and I am honored that he has written the Foreword to this book. Those who regularly read the *Publisher's Letter* in *Modern Healthcare* are familiar the influence of his inspiration. I am grateful for the wisdom he shares with us every week and for his friendship.

I would also like to thank David Burda, editor, and Fawn Lopez, associate publisher, of *Modern Healthcare* for the pleasure of working with them and for their commitment to the award program.

You can tell a lot about a corporate culture by interacting with its people over time. One does not need to read Sodexho's annual report to know that this company invests in relationships; or that excellence, respect, and integrity are driving values. Everyone at Sodexho Health Care Services with whom I have worked for more than a decade has consistently demonstrated these expectations and qualities. I would especially like to thank Lynne Adame, Carol Ganci, and Jay Marvin for their roles in making this relationship enjoyable and rewarding.

I would also like to acknowledge that employees of Sodexho Health Care Services are disqualified from entering the award competition. Yet, over the years, entries have been submitted by Sodexho clients, most often by executives wanting to recognize the merits of a department's performance. I made the independent decision to include some of these profiles. Neither Sodexho nor *Modern Healthcare* has exerted influence on the selection of entries in this book or other editorial or production decisions. I am grateful for their confidence and for the opportunity to write about the program they co-sponsor.

The profiles in this book were first composed by more than 130 different individuals; these are their stories. My challenge was to organize the material and retell it in a way that did not compromise the factual integrity or distort the "voice" of the author. Fortunately I had a couple of wonderful advisors.

Thanks to Wendy Husser, who is the executive editor of a prestigious medical journal and my neighbor. Wendy read the entire manuscript three weeks before it was sent to the printer and offered edits and instructive comments. She was so generous with her time and most gracious in her support.

ACKNOWLEDGMENTS

I also want to thank Cynthia Sucher. Cynthia provided me with valuable suggestions and advice on numerous occasions. I will never forget one return phone call from her in response to an inquiry. She answered my question and then calmly told me that she had to hang up and leave the office because a hurricane was about to hit Orlando.

Thanks to so many who have contributed in various ways to this book: Saundra Atwood, Kris Baird, Bridget Baird, Judith Calhoun, Mark Dziewior, John Eudes, Jay Greene, Steve Hillestad, Joyce Jensen, Scott MacStravic, John Stavros, Jim Szczepaniak, and Laurie Wilshusen.

Thanks to Bill Sosin, who painstakingly laid out this book and maintained admirable humor and patience throughout the process. And thanks to Terry Ernsberger for the great cover design. Terry is also responsible for creating Greystone Interactive's wonderful Web site, and it is always a delight to work with him.

Generosity is the term that most appropriately describes what I discovered soon after I undertook this project and personal circumstances caused an interruption. To all who extended generous support, encouragement, contribution, and patience, I thank you.

Kristine Peterson
Editor, *The Spirit of Excellence*
President, Greystone Interactive
December 2004

THE SPIRIT OF EXCELLENCE

Please proceed to each chapter for a Table of Contents.

FOREWORD

F OR TWELVE YEARS, MODERN HEALTHCARE has been a proud co-sponsor of the annual Sodexho Spirit of Excellence award program. Our mission from the start has been to recognize the best programs and practices being implemented by health care organizations. I am told by those who judge this competition that it is challenging to select a relatively few as the winning entries because so many projects are deserving of recognition. This book honors the many organizations that have demonstrated ambitions to excel and achieve their visions.

The wide range of projects in this book makes a statement about how health care organizations view their roles as providers, employers, and stakeholders in the communities they serve. In addition to the institutions that have taken patient, resident or employee satisfaction to soaring heights, there are numerous heart-warming projects that reveal the insight and creativity of individuals who see opportunities to fill unmet needs and take action. You will discover a hospital system that is bringing the tradition of storytelling into the inpatient setting to help patients and families capture healing moments. You will read about nurses who invite local politicians to "walk a mile in our shoes" to better understand the essential roles nurses play in assuring quality of care. You will learn how nursing homes are transforming food services into dining experiences that residents look forward to. You will sense the spirit that unites individuals in achieving a common goal, whether it is building ramps so discharged patients can gain access to their homes, improving processes so patients can gain quicker access to emergency services, or developing accessible apartment complexes so disabled persons can live independently.

> *The wide range of projects in this book makes a statement about **how health care organizations** view their roles as providers, employers, and stakeholders in the **communities they serve.***

The late Karl Bays, the legendary leader of American Hospital Supply, used to say, "Healthcare is a business, but the business is about taking care of people." I was reminded of the wisdom of his words as I read the stories in this book. Health care is a complicated business and we should never forget how lucky we all are to work among exceptional people who invest their knowledge and energies to heal broken hearts and mend broken bones. The content of this book is all about performance; the subtext is all about people. People taking care of people.

Sodexho Health Care Services deserves tremendous praise for conceiving and funding this prestigious award competition. By doing so, this respected company affirms its passion for excellence and the commitment it extends to meet the needs and exceed the expectations of the customers it serves. Kristine Peterson is to be commended for doing something that should have been done a long time ago—relating the remarkable stories that have inspired all of us who have been fortunate to read Sodexho Spirit of Excellence entries each year.

The message is clear: Great things happen when organizations and individuals commit to excellence.

Chuck Lauer
Publisher, *Modern Healthcare*
December 2004

INTRODUCTION

THIS BOOK IS TITLED THE SPIRIT OF EXCELLENCE, for two reasons. One, "Spirit of Excellence" is the name of the award program co-sponsored by Sodexho Health Care Services and *Modern Healthcare*. Each year the Spirit of Excellence awards spotlight innovative programs that contribute to excellence. This book is a compendium of the excellent projects submitted to this competition.

The other reason this book is named THE SPIRIT OF EXCELLENCE is quite simple; excellence cannot be achieved without spirit. Spirit is the animating principle that gives life to physical organisms—and to organizations. As such, spirit is vapor-like. It does not necessarily condense when put on paper, but it is there and you will be able to sense it.

Spirit is what makes a team of individuals unite around a shared goal and invest their efforts to lift performance. The etymology of the word, spirit is from the Latin *spirare* and means "to blow, to breathe." I think of spirit as the wind beneath the wings of every project in this book.

When you read my comments that follow the profile of Huron Valley–Sinai Hospital I hope you will understand that this whimsical example of spirit is an indication that there is more to each of the stories in this book than meets the eye. When I spoke with Heather Mac Donald of Capital Health District Authority in Nova Scotia to learn more about the Critical Care Council, she told me one of the reasons they expanded the scope of their care to families of ICU patients was because of what they read in the Bible. No, her reference was not specific to the inspired word of God, but to the inspired words of family members as they recorded their feelings on the pages of a Bible that was left in the ICU waiting room. These are not comments that people write on patient satisfaction surveys. Hearing the silent cries of people who are dealing with illness and loss are vitally important if we are going to make connections that are meaningful to our customers. To do that, we have to stay close to our customers; see them, hear them, touch them, smell them, and taste the bitterness and sweetness of their experiences.

If ... someone is inspired to say, 'We can do that too!' the book has served a purpose.

THE SPIRIT OF EXCELLENCE award program recognizes initiatives that demonstrate excellence in customer service (Service Spirit), improve quality, safety, and performance (Quality Spirit), build workforce commitment (Team Spirit), and meet the needs of communities through education and outreach (Community Spirit). It was challenging to organize these stories into four discrete categories because there is wide overlap. We created nine chapters, and there are many profiles included in one chapter that could have been included in a different chapter. You will discover that some of the stories are very similar. Despite the similarities, there is something worthwhile in an approach, an idea, or an outcome that caused me to believe that each story added value.

All of these projects are "best practices" although not in the conventional sense of the word. Basically, these profiles are about projects that were submitted for review in an award competition. They represent feelings of ownership and pride. There may, for example, be inventory control systems that are more sophisticated than the one implemented by Vernon Manor, but I believe this particular example points out a couple of important things: 1) someone or a team of individuals *took the initiative to improve* a process because there was an evident need to do so, and 2) small, seemingly insignificant ideas may add up to big savings or improved satisfaction. Although we don't know how much money Vernon Manor has saved since stamping its identity on linens, it has evidently had an impact.

While we can never learn whether a butterfly's fluttering in Brazil causes hurricanes in Florida, it is clear that what happens within individual departments can affect an entire organization. The dietary director at Lindsborg Community Hospital decided to do something about food waste. Karna Peterson and her team created "Healthy Fast Food to Go." This innovative service responds to unmet needs in the community and contributes revenue to the hospital. Another example is found in Gibson General Hospital. Finding no comparable, affordable database to meet the benchmarking needs of rural health care providers, Sharon Doran and her team created "Apples to Apples," a service that now benefits 90 rural health care providers across the country. Karna and Sharon each saw a need, recognized an opportunity, and took the initiative—unaware at the time of the implications.

A single success catalyzed the emergency department at Cape Canaveral Hospital and initiated improvements that caused satisfaction and spirits to soar. Digital clocks installed outside of each exam room in Duncan Regional Hospital's emergency department serve to remind staff how long it has been since someone interacted with a patient. It is termed an "elegant" solution because of its simplicity and positive impact. Carondelet St. Joseph's Hospital's "Ruby Slippers" and OSU & Harding Behavioral Healthcare and Medicine's discoveries about pain management are other examples worthy of note. It can be argued that "everything counts," and small things can make big differences.

There are many more examples in this book that relate to the "Butterfly Effect." Organizations driven by excellence and powered by spirit are always seeking ways to improve. Providence Centralia Hospital assigned all departments the responsibility of improving a work process that acted as a barrier to providing excellent customer service. They sought small projects that could be implemented in nine months. Incremental improvement is better than inaction. "Big, hairy, audacious goals" (BHAGs) are great, but sometimes BHAGs are anathema to initiative.

COMPARED WITH "SERVICE" PROJECTS that were submitted to the Sodexho award program a decade ago, organizational initiatives that are implemented today are much more serious, pervasive, and far-reaching. We've moved beyond thinking of customer service as training people to be nice, and we now have tools that are much more sophisticated than we had then. One tool, patient satisfaction measurement and the capability to benchmark, has had a phenomenal impact on improvement and initiative. As Conemaugh Memorial Medical Center writes, *"If someone had asked us a couple of years ago how our patients rated Conemaugh Memorial Medical Center, we would have said, "Great!" Those were the days when we used a homemade survey tool that asked patients to agree or disagree with our satisfaction assumptions. Of course, anything approximating agreement was alright, in which case, 98% of our patients were happy."* When its first benchmarking report came in after the hospital contracted with a national firm to conduct satisfaction research, everyone was shocked to learn the hospital ranked in the 22nd percentile. Conemaugh got over the disbelief and did not stand still. The hospital's turnaround earned them a Spirit of Excellence award. You will read a similar account of how customer feedback changed the orientations and practices

INTRODUCTION

of a pediatric oncology nursing unit at Hackensack University Medical Center. These are great examples of how the bellow of customer feedback causes wings to flutter.

Giving customers a "voice" has done a lot to improve service. And benchmarking has contributed to wiping out the TGE (That's Good Enough) malaise. It is a blessing, but benchmarking can be a curse. It is easy to overlook that when you are ranked in the 90th percentile, this does not mean 9 of 10 customers are satisfied with your performance.

To make another point: Nordstrom has not achieved its strength in the retail sector because 95% of its customers are satisfied. Nordstrom is the giant it is because 30% of its customers walk out of the store with a desire to tell a story—to tell someone about what makes shopping at Nordstrom so satisfying. Although I have no idea what values are accurate to relate in that example, I hope the point was made.

Organizations that move from the 10th percentile to the 95th percentile certainly deserve applause, but so do those that do not have major turnarounds to report. What I find to be impressive is the organization that moves the needle in the direction of "very satisfied" customers. Griffin Hospital offers valuable perspectives on this.

Organizations that succeed are aware of how their performance compares to similar organizations, but they push the envelope because they have a champion mindset; they are often competing against their own personal best, and they are not looking to copy anyone.

Metrics other than customer satisfaction are used to gauge the success of projects in this book. The full range of criterion includes dimensions such as quality benchmarks, productivity, cost savings, and staff retention; the "what if" dimensions relating to prevention of illness, mistakes or litigation; the outcome dimensions relating to market share, revenue, and margin; and other important dimensions that defy quantification, such as improving the quality of life, the quality of dying, or the quality of caring simply because it is the right thing to do. When you read the profiles of Windy Hill Village, St. Bernardine Medical Center, Walton Rehabilitation Hospital, and others, it will be obvious that there is always a return on investment.

Other than a reference made in this Introduction, I have not identified the winners of Sodexho Spirit of Excellence awards in this book. Articles about the winners have appeared in *Modern Healthcare* and you can read those online at: www.modernhealthcare.com.

The second volume of THE SPIRIT OF EXCELLENCE is currently in production, and it will include many more stories about how health care organizations are achieving service, quality, and satisfaction. I hope you will find these editions to be helpful in lifting the performance of your organization. I also hope to be able to include your stories in the future.

I have been honored to help recognize the contributions of many people. If, after reading one of the profiles, someone is inspired to say, "We can do that too!" this book has served another important purpose.

Kristine Peterson

CHAPTER 1
SERVICE EXCELLENCE

SERVICE EXCELLENCE

Advocate Health Care, the largest integrated health care system in metropolitan Chicago, embarked on a journey to live up to its values by dramatically improving patient satisfaction scores across the system of eight hospitals and more than two hundred sites of care. Advocate knew it would be no small undertaking to move the system as a whole from its 23rd percentile ranking in a national database toward its target of achieving the 95th percentile. Within two years, Advocate Health Care had achieved this goal.

Advocate Health Care's mission, values and philosophy (MVP) assure that we will provide patients and families with superior service. Thus, we adopted a strategy known as "Service Breakthrough" to improve service delivery at all Advocate sites of care and aligned physician practices. Two years of relentless effort and steady improvement followed. Our strategies included:

Start at the Top. After reviewing patient satisfaction scores and hearing from the system's site chief executives about their roles in leading the initiative, Advocate's board of directors added "service excellence" as a standing agenda item at every board meeting. Our senior leaders devoted an entire retreat to service excellence. After the retreat, our learning continued as we hosted presentations by outside speakers, scheduled site visits, and researched best practices. At every senior management meeting, we reviewed the status of improvement efforts and identified ways to leverage successful initiatives and learn from tactics that did not yield results.

Create a Service Excellence Policy. Our human resources department developed a new policy that holds all associates accountable for delivering outstanding service and empowers managers to act when associates are not living up to those expectations. The service excellence policy defines Advocate's service strategy and explains both acceptable and unacceptable behaviors. The purpose of this policy was to help associates align performance with Advocate's service expectations.

Develop Performance Standards. Most Advocate associates were familiar with the organization's five values of compassion, equality, excellence, partnership, and stewardship. But knowing what the values are and actually living up to those values are two different things. We developed a set of behavioral standards that translated Advocate's MVP into concrete actions. These performance standards apply to all associates—at every level—within Advocate.

Identify Quick Hits. Advocate's senior leadership, and representatives from all sites who participated on a team, agreed to a set of system-wide "quick hits" that were implemented throughout the organization.

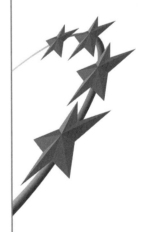

*Advocate
Health Care*

Oak Brook, Ill.

These relatively simple tasks had an immediate impact on patient satisfaction and included the following:

- visits to all new admissions by a nursing manager
- follow-up calls to all discharged patients by nurse caregivers
- service recovery allowances of up to $250
- dry-erase communications boards in all patient rooms
- key word and phrase usage
- reminders to notify patients of our commitment to protect their privacy
- responsibility for answering call lights shared by everyone

Benchmark Internally and Externally. Advocate created a new educational series titled, "Service Breakthrough Best Practices Showcase," which periodically allows departments to present successful programs and practices to their counterparts throughout the system. A section was created on Advocate's Intranet that contains ideas and insights that can help save time and jump-start success by implementing proven best practices.

Introduce Service Scripts. Advocate developed scripts for associates to use during interactions with patients. These scripts are designed to ensure that each contact with the patient results in a positive impression. Even in the most common situations, a well-crafted statement is memorable and will leave a lasting impression. A collection of scripts, to reduce variation in our service, provides both actions and words for critical patient/customer interactions. By making scripts a part of their everyday routines, associates can exceed patients' expectations.

Train Leaders and Associates. All managers received 80 hours of training related to building associate satisfaction and customer satisfaction. A core curriculum of five courses is mandatory for all new managers to complete within their first six months of employment as Advocate leaders. Additional courses were designed to help leaders understand their patient satisfaction results and identify specific improvement areas. The organizational development department revamped Advocate's orientation program for new associates. The new program is called "Training Camp for Advocate Champions" and it has strengthened the emphasis on service excellence. The coaches even developed scripts to reduce service variation in how messages are communicated during orientation. This helps to ensure that every new employee has a clear understanding of our commitment and expectations.

Encourage Service Recovery. The task force assigned the responsibility for service recovery outlined a simple process for all associates to follow. Advocate adopted five steps for service recovery. These are as follow: 1) listen

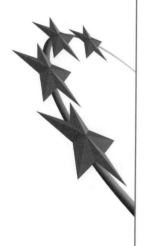

***Advocate
Health Care***

Oak Brook, Ill.

to the patient/customer and own the problem, 2) apologize/empathize, 3) respond by fixing the problem, 4) express thanks, and 5) follow-up.

Celebrate Service Heroes and Milestones. Service excellence is celebrated throughout the system. Advocate's service heroes—those associates who have done something beyond the scope of their job responsibilities to meet the needs of customers—are recognized for making a real difference in our efforts to improve patient satisfaction.

Advocate started at the top but without thousands of dedicated people on the front-line of care, we would not have achieved success. Service Breakthrough empowered us to break through barriers that prevented us from achieving the performance we aspired to deliver. We climbed from the 23rd percentile to the 95th percentile in patient satisfaction within two years. Our performance reflects our faith-based mission of caring that has been the foundation of our heritage for over 100 years.

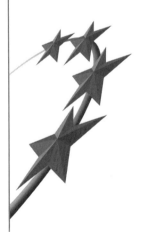

Advocate
Health Care
Oak Brook, Ill.

A commitment to excellence and a vision of becoming the region's premier employer were driving forces that led to DuBois Regional Medical Center being named one of the "Top 100 Workplaces in Pennsylvania." The organization's leaders embraced the goal of transforming the culture to reflect the values and principles of the service excellence initiative and extended their support to the process. By engaging employees in improvement efforts, DuBois executed its bold strategy and succeeded in building community and employee confidence about the future direction of the medical center.

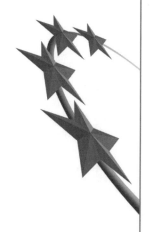

DuBois Regional Medical Center

DuBois, Pa.

DuBois Regional Medical Center is the sole health care provider in a large rural area of Pennsylvania. Although the organization had been strong financially, we had begun to lose market share in some service areas. DuBois also had begun to experience high turnover and struggled to recruit nurses and other health care workers. The entire senior management team committed to the values, principles, and behaviors of our Customer Service Excellence Initiative (CSEI). The executives realized that we would need to spend money to make money and committed the resources needed to assure adequate staffing, training, equipment, and leadership development.

We knew it would take a top-down approach to truly make substantial changes in our performance, so the vice president of patient services spearheaded the CSEI. After investigating strategies that were successful in other hospitals, a team of leaders visited Baptist Hospital in Pensacola, Fla., to learn more about their success in customer service. These leaders became the founding members of our steering committee. We created a strategic plan that focused on two major elements: 1) implementing customer service teams to engage all levels of employees in improvement efforts, and 2) fostering a culture of customer service to transform the way our leaders and employees value and serve our patients and each other.

The first major strategy involved starting numerous teams. The Measurement Team implemented a patient satisfaction measurement process to ensure that customer feedback became the driving force for improvement. The Standards Team developed core behaviors for all employees to practice each day. A Celebrations Team implemented activities to recognize customer service excellence and encourage everyone to "catch people doing things right."

The Service Recovery Team implemented strategies to help employees take corrective action when patient expectations are not met. The 'What's Bugging You?' Team uncovered barriers to service excellence and removed them. A team in the emergency department dramatically turned around patient satisfaction, patient wait times and other key performance measures.

The Inpatient Satisfaction Team helped all departments improve patient satisfaction by focusing on priorities identified in satisfaction survey results. The Outpatient Satisfaction Team implemented customer-focused strategies, both inside the hospital and in the community. One priority was making sure signage to our hospital from the major highways was directional.

The second major strategy was transforming our culture. We focused on five key issues designed to:

- improve clinical quality by hiring a dedicated performance improvement manager and a vice president of medical affairs, as well as investing in technology to provide data to drive improvements;

- provide intensive leadership development and employee training;

- improve the human resource management systems and become the region's premier employer for health care;

- demonstrate leadership commitment to the strategic priorities of high service, high quality, best people, and low cost through daily decisions and actions;

- build support for patient care by removing barriers that prevent effective work; and

- celebrate the great work that is done each day.

The core philosophy that we embraced at the outset of the CSEI was a promise to take good care of our employees and they, in turn, would do the same for our patients. Leadership development was necessary to help managers communicate the values, model the behaviors, and build the performance of employees. A work team created leadership standards of performance to define the expected practices. A leadership scorecard that links recognition and reward to CSEI goals is now used during annual performance reviews. We have proven that strong leadership at all levels of the organization is essential to success.

A second major change in employee relations was leadership support of employee work by focusing on operations, resource management, training and development, and hiring practices. Leaders began making clinical rounds and helping staff with problems. Recognizing that many problems are related to short staffing, we decided to develop staffing resources through our workforce development initiative. A group of leaders and employees began working with the five school districts in our region to promote health careers. We educated guidance counselors, created a Health Career Hotline, instituted job shadowing and student volunteer programs, developed middle school after-hours enrichment programs, and started a Medical Explorers Post. As a result, some 60 RNs have graduated from our scholarship program

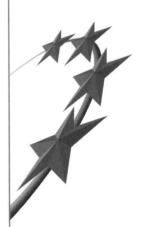

DuBois Regional Medical Center

DuBois, Pa.

in the last three years and now are employed here. We received the Hospital Association of Pennsylvania Achievement Award for our accomplishments in workforce development.

A final and imperative focus has been on creating a positive, healthy work environment. To accomplish this, we do the following:

- respond to employee satisfaction results and make improvements

- recognize, reward, and celebrate individuals, teams and departments

- improve physical work environments

- assure adequate, competent staffing

- work to improve physician–staff relations

- invest in technology to reduce workload

- improve patient care and employee work environments

- use CSEI values as hiring criteria

- engage staff in improvement initiatives

During the five years of our Customer Service Excellence Initiative, the teams and culture-building strategies have changed but the goals never have. Everyone is now focused on exceeding the 95th percentile in patient satisfaction and growing our volumes and market share. Everything we do and the decisions we make are focused on what is best for our patients and our employees.

We recently conducted another employee satisfaction survey and ranked the second highest organization in the database. Great improvements were noted in areas such as employee confidence in leadership and the direction the organization is heading. Employees are satisfied that our priorities are focused in the right areas and that we maintain a commitment to excellent patient care. Our clinical quality measures are consistently high with many exceeding national benchmarks and our technological investments are paying off. We were named one of the "Top 100 Workplaces in Pennsylvania!" We are committed to stay the course and accomplish even more.

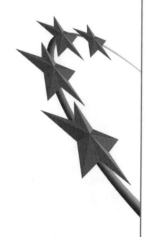

DuBois Regional Medical Center

DuBois, Pa.

Several years ago, Parkview Hospital opened the doors of two new hospitals, Parkview North Hospital and the adjoining Orthopaedic Hospital at Parkview North. Reasoning that it would be more important to focus on quality assurance, rather than customer service until the new operation was running smoothly, the suggestion was made to set patient satisfaction goals around the 75th percentile. Understanding the undesired consequence of setting low targets, as well as having a keen appreciation for the symbiotic characteristics of quality and service, Parkview leaders immediately dismissed the notion and identified the 90th percentile as the desired performance target for patient satisfaction. Their ambitious expectations were exceeded when Parkview North was ranked in the 99th percentile in all three service areas (inpatient, outpatient and emergency) in the first quarter of operation.

Together Parkview North Hospital and Orthopaedic Hospital at Parkview North (hereafter referred to as Parkview North), offer 65 inpatient beds (medical/surgical, orthopaedics, obstetrics), eight operating rooms, an emergency department, and outpatient services. Parkview North is located on the north side of Fort Wayne where competition for market share is high because Parkview's primary competitor built a new hospital two miles away. Determined to create a staff culture that would place the highest importance on exceeding customer expectations, the chief operating officer and director of nursing developed a Quality Customer Service Plan (QCSP) that adapted customer service and quality improvement principles from the Disney Institute, Florida Power & Light and Parkview Hospital's existing program.

During planning retreats, the management team created service principles.These principles are courtesy, accountability, customer focus, innovation, and teamwork. The plan was later reviewed and approved by the Customer Service Committee of Parkview Health, the system entity to which we belong.

Understanding customer/patient expectations and measuring satisfaction were integral parts of the plan. Emphasis was placed on building a strong customer service orientation among all employees. Regular recognition and feedback that encouraged and rewarded desired customer service behaviors and outcomes were also deemed important. Our service strategies yielded the following initiatives and services:

Customer Service Representative. A full-time customer service representative is responsible for monitoring customer satisfaction, working with managers to address customer concerns, providing service recovery, and identifying areas for improvement. All patients receive a visit from this representative.

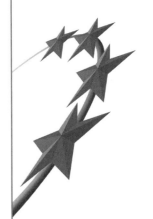

Parkview
North
Hospital

Fort Wayne, Ind.

Quality Service Matrix. The most innovative and effective aspect of the Quality Customer Service Plan is a matrix that is used by each department to develop its own QCSP. This matrix allows the manager and his/her employees to evaluate three major care delivery systems (employees, facilities and process) in the context of the our five service quality principles.

Adopt-An-Area. All employees are involved in keeping the physical environment looking its best. Areas are judged monthly and the winning department receives lunch, compliments of Parkview North.

Leadership and Department Meetings. All management and department meetings are required to include "quality customer service" as an agenda item. Volunteers also receive training in customer service.

Surveys/Comment Cards. Satisfaction surveys are routed to managers for review and follow-up. Results are shared with staff and appropriate phone calls are made to address any described concerns. Comment cards are available to gather information regarding service while the patient is in the facility. Follow up is done regarding concerns that are noted.

Patient Focus Groups. Held four times a year and facilitated by the chief operating officer, these groups include former patients who are invited to a dinner meeting to share their comments regarding their care.

Staff Quality Service Award. Employees nominate co-workers who have excelled in customer service. The monthly winner is recognized with a photo, certificate, and $50 gift.

PEOPLE Awards for Staff Excellence. Co-workers and supervisors give PEOPLE Awards to employees who show exemplary customer service. Management is reminded to use this vehicle to recognize staff. At milestones of 10, 25, and 50 awards, employees receive a gift.

Letters/PEOPLE Awards. Staff members who are complimented by name on a patient survey or comment card are sent a letter of recognition and listed in the internal newsletter. They also receive a PEOPLE Award. Physicians who are complimented by name on a satisfaction survey are sent a letter from the COO. They also receive a PEOPLE Award and are recognized in the medical staff newsletter.

Staff Focus Groups. Members of the staff are randomly selected to participate in focus groups, which are facilitated by the COO three times a year. They are asked for input on how to improve our service.

A recent employee opinion survey reflected high mean scores for Parkview North in areas related to quality customer service and employee satisfaction.

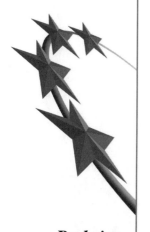

Parkview North Hospital

Fort Wayne, Ind.

We earned the highest mean scores among ten Parkview Health facilities in the following areas:

- Employees care about providing excellent service – 96.6

- Customer satisfaction is one of our most important measures of success – 94.5

- My department works hard to improve customer satisfaction – 94.1

- My manager treats me with dignity and respect – 94.0

Parkview North scored in the 99th percentile in all three areas of service (inpatient, outpatient and emergency) for its first quarter results.

Parkview Health contracted with a market research firm to conduct a blind telephone survey. Among the eight area hospitals mentioned in the "overall quality of care" category, Parkview North had the highest mean scores in inpatient, outpatient, and emergency.

Setting ambitious goals at the outset simply matched our staff's ambitions to perform, exceed and excel.

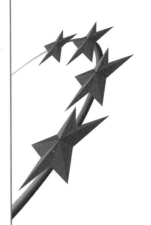

Parkview North Hospital

Fort Wayne, Ind.

In the early 1990s, the market area served by Thomas Hospital experienced explosive growth. This growth introduced opportunities and challenges, both of which were addressed when hospital leaders presented annual goals to the board of directors. The first goal was to attain the 95th percentile in patient satisfaction by delivering excellent customer service. The second goal was to meet or exceed financial targets. Believing these two goals were inextricably related, the hospital launched its campaign to improve service and financial performance. Within one year, Thomas Hospital moved from a fiscal year loss of $2.9 million to a $3 million gain while consistently exceeding customer expectations.

For many years, Thomas Hospital was a small town hospital and provided primary care to residents of the community. Our mission reflected the communities we served; neighbors taking care of neighbors. Patients with serious medical problems went to larger urban hospitals.

Once Baldwin County began to experience tremendous growth, our leaders realized patients would no longer be satisfied receiving the small town care that the hospital family had delivered for many years. The mission of Thomas Hospital changed to reflect this growth and change. We adopted a new mission statement, pledging that Thomas Hospital would be "the premier provider of health care in Baldwin County and surrounding areas." By using advanced skills and technology, Thomas Hospital would "improve the health status and quality of life." Most importantly, patients would receive their care "in an atmosphere of compassion, sensitivity and respect."

The goal was to provide medical services that would allow residents of Baldwin County to have their health care needs met locally. New doctors began moving in and the hospital went from 400 employees to 980 employees in just ten years. It was a decade filled with challenges, both financial and operational, at a time when our ability to make a cultural shift was crucial in determining our future destiny.

As we began to view our mission and role differently, it was natural that we would begin to view our structure and organizational priorities differently as well. Our first step was to turn the organizational chart upside down. Management named the hospital's five customer groups—patients, employees, physicians, volunteers, and the community—and placed these groups at the top of the chart. The board of directors and administration were at the bottom of the chart to demonstrate servant leadership.

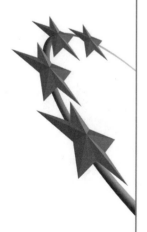

Thomas Hospital

Fairhope, Ala.

Administration appointed a director of customer service who, along with a core team of employees, created and implemented customer service initiatives. The hospital adopted "Quest for the Best" as its customer service slogan. The goal of this program was to achieve the 95th percentile or better in patient satisfaction.

Employees were asked to submit examples of behaviors that personified great customer service. Once those behaviors were clarified, we focused on one behavior each month and produced a series of videos and posters to emphasize the service behaviors. Hospital employees wrote the scripts and acted in the videos. For example, one employee wrote a script using a *"Survivor"* theme borrowed from the popular television program to reinforce teamwork. The cast of employee actors went to a public beach to act out the skit. Videos were distributed to all departments. In addition to the videos, posters were placed throughout the hospital. Physicians, employees and employees' children were featured in the posters that served to remind everyone of the behavior of the month. We developed and implemented other customer service improvements and initiatives:

Service Recovery Program. Employees may purchase an item in the hospital's gift shop to enhance patient or visitor satisfaction.

Lullaby. The hospital's foundation commissioned a local symphonic quartet to record an original lullaby that is played every time a baby is born.

Customer Service Pledge. New employees sign a customer service pledge to confirm their commitment to uphold the customer service standards.

Birthday Bash. Our president/CEO hosts a monthly birthday party and holds informal discussions with those who are celebrating a birthday during that month.

Hospitality Assistants. Hospitality assistants deliver food trays, respond to special food requests, retrieve and deliver movies from a video library and deliver e-greetings (e-mails sent through the hospital's Web site).

Notepads for Patients. Notepads imprinted *"Questions I'd like to ask ..."* are available in all patient rooms to encourage patients and family members to write down questions they want to ask their doctors.

Employee Fun. To foster a creative culture and community involvement, we sponsored employee appreciation events including: a Cajun Cook-off to raise money for the Heart Association; an Iron Bowl Fish Fry in conjunction with a local food drive; a Follies Night featuring skits by hospital departments to raise money for the American Cancer Society.

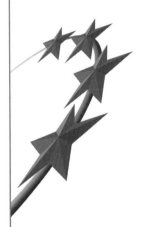

Thomas Hospital

Fairhope, Ala.

Commitment to Improve Communication. A video is produced quarterly to highlight events and provide updates on hospital-related news. The employee newsletter has been expanded and redesigned. Each year, the president/CEO asks department heads/managers to complete the following sentence in writing: *"If I were President of Thomas Hospital, I would..."*

Employees serve on the core team for a period of one year. This term of involvement helps to involve as many employees as possible in the Quest for the Best program and to generate fresh ideas. Each director is asked to include a customer service goal in his/her annual department's goals.

The hospital has made it a point to let the public in on its efforts to improve customer service. A glass case located next to the main elevators displays quarterly satisfaction scores by department. Articles about customer service are published in the hospital's quarterly publications and monthly employee newsletters.

After the launch of Quest for the Best, the hospital's patient satisfaction ranking, which had hovered in the low-to-mid 80s for years, was in the 99th percentile for three straight quarters. Each quarter since, the hospital has achieved its overall goal of ranking in the 95th percentile or better. We celebrate with "95-cent Day," wherein a meal in the cafeteria costs only 95-cents when this goal is met. Quarterly pizza parties and banners honor departments with the highest and the most improved patient satisfaction scores.

The hospital also has achieved financial success. Within one year, we went from a $2.9 million loss to a $3 million gain. We do not believe this is coincidental: Quest for the Best became an organizational mindset and an individual commitment, empowering us to achieve great outcomes.

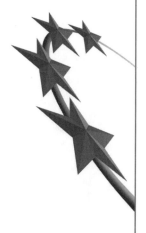

Thomas Hospital

Fairhope, Ala.

The outlook for Conemaugh Memorial Medical Center was not positive several years ago. Inpatient satisfaction scores were in the 22nd percentile, $2 million per month was lost in operations and market share was slipping. Now, the medical center enjoys soaring patient satisfaction scores, national recognition for clinical outcomes, solid volumes, and financial strength. Conemaugh Memorial achieved this impressive success by listening to and involving experts with the experience to guide organizational change—patients, physicians and employees.

If someone had asked us a couple of years ago how our patients rated Conemaugh Memorial Medical Center, we would have said, "Great!" Those were the days when we used a homemade survey tool that asked patients to agree or disagree with our satisfaction assumptions. Anything approximating agreement was alright; in which case, 98% of our patients were happy. Yet, if we were doing so well, why was our financial outlook so bleak? Why was our employee morale so low? Why was our market share eroding?

At that time, our focus was on our financial status. It had to be. We were losing, on average, $2 million a month from operations. We had already redesigned every process imaginable by following the recommendations of a consulting firm that is recognized for its success in health care re-engineering. When losses continued, we decided that redesign wasn't enough.

Leaders identified a triad on which we were to focus. Clinical excellence, service excellence, and cost effectiveness became the top three priorities for direction-setting activities. No longer was the sole focus to be financial. To guide us in the right direction, someone suggested that we ask the experts—our customers. As we began listening to patients, we considered other untapped group of experts—our employees and physicians.

We formed a Hospitality Team to help steer us in the right direction. During the initial months, foundations were set behind-the-scenes. The team developed Golden Rules—fourteen standards of behavior all employees were to exemplify. As we began to educate staff and managers about the Golden Rules, we also began to reward those who demonstrated them. Our Gold Star program has been a huge success. Staff physicians and volunteers, as well as employees, are eligible to be nominated for these awards that are presented monthly at management meetings.

Concurrent with the birth of our Gold Star program, our performance improvement (PI) program was reorganized, providing yet another opportunity for employees to join teams and use their creativity to make improvements and solve problems. We implemented a new structure that enables departments to report PI activities on a rotating basis every month.

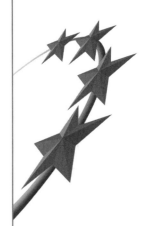

Conemaugh Memorial Medical Center

Johnstown, Pa.

This allows each department to showcase successes and request input from other departments to help with weak areas.

We understood we needed to benchmark our performance against national standards. We contracted with a national firm to conduct satisfaction research. When the first report came in, no one could believe that we were in the 22nd percentile compared to our peers! Immediately, several PI teams began to use satisfaction data to identify process improvement opportunities within their departments.

We decided to visit another facility to learn how we could do even better. This site visit showed us that we were indeed headed in the right direction; we had many of the tools in place to be successful. We also learned that we really needed to focus more on the patients. We knew it all along, but the financial focus seemed to still creep to the forefront now and then.

An expanded structure was developed to support the organization-wide changes. Nine multidisciplinary teams used satisfaction data to facilitate broad-based organizational change. Thanks to our Inpatient Team, we now make post-discharge courtesy calls, send thank-you cards, and have enhanced our infant bereavement process. The Leadership Development Team completed an assessment to determine the educational needs of the organization's leaders. These needs were identified, not only by the leaders themselves, but also by staff they manage.

The Hospitality Team developed the Golden Rules into behavioral standards. The Employee Satisfaction Team is expanding the Gold Star program to improve employee satisfaction and purchasing equipment for a new Employee Wellness Center. Our Physician Satisfaction Team is about to celebrate a first—we're sending out a physician satisfaction survey.

Inpatient satisfaction scores for a recent quarter ranked us at the 92nd percentile. The other two elements of our triad have improved as well. We were recognized for clinical excellence when named a "Top 100 Heart Hospital" and a "Top 100 Orthopaedic Hospital." As for the financial aspect, admissions have increased 6% over last year. The monthly loss from operations is now a gain of $370,000 per month, on average.

The consultants told us to redesign. We did. We still lost money and our performance didn't improve. We then involved the real experts in our improvement process. We listened and responded to our patients and staff. As a result, we've witnessed improvements in clinical excellence, financial performance, and customer satisfaction. We learned that listening to customers really delivers results.

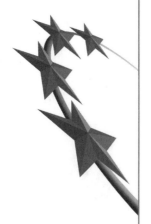

Conemaugh Memorial Medical Center

Johnstown, Pa.

A few years ago, Huron Valley–Sinai Hospital experienced stagnant volumes, recruitment and retention difficulties, and financial distress. It was challenging to keep a positive service outlook amid the many competing priorities. The 153-bed hospital now enjoys solid financial performance, exceptionally satisfied patients, a staff vacancy rate of less than 6%, and a team that plays together.

Baseball great, Babe Ruth once said, "The way a team plays as a whole determines its success. You may have the greatest bunch of individual stars in the world but if they don't play together, the team won't be worth a dime." At Huron Valley–Sinai Hospital, we have achieved great results by setting clear expectations and working as a team to exceed customer expectations. We play to win. We demonstrate our commitment by focusing on the following areas:

Persistent in Obtaining Customer Feedback. We ask patients and families what we can do to satisfy their needs, improve their satisfaction or answer their questions. We listen to our customers, patients, and families and make changes to our processes to improve their experience while in our care. Customer satisfaction data are reviewed carefully and shared with all managers and employees.

Insistent on Recognizing Employees. To immediately reinforce customer service behaviors, we give our employees a variety of $20 gift certificates known as Spot Awards. We also reward employees who are nominated for excellent customer service and are chosen by the Customer Service Team to be recognized. These recipients may receive up to $200. We have a Wall of Fame listing those recognized for service excellence each month. Each department also has a bulletin board that can be used to display customer service information and recognize employees.

Consistent in Service Delivery. Erratic performance means some customers receive great service and others do not. Our aim is to deliver great service consistently. We developed a Customer Service University that is available to all employees. Managers continuously coach employees to help them achieve their performance potential. We listen to our employees and note changes that need to be made. We also have a "Wednesday Morning Workout" e-mail that is shared with all employees. This e-mail consists of motivational customer service information and ideas to promote service excellence.

The administrative coordinator of customer service visits each unit every week to discuss customer service. She takes a cheerleader doll, appropriately named "Valley," and a basket filled with candy to share with all. Valley is more than mascot. She has assumed a position on our team.

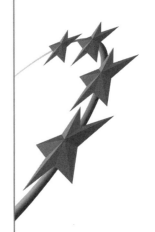

Huron Valley–
Sinai Hospital

Commerce, Mich.

Our employees are aware of the important positions they play on the team. Huron Valley–Sinai Hospital has winning spirit and it shows!

EDITOR'S NOTE: During the final stages of editing, I called Dot Kempf, the administrative director of customer service at Huron Valley-Sinai Hospital. Because it was necessary to condense some of the profiles, I wanted to confirm that we had captured the essence of the story in the edited version that appears above. I hesitatingly asked whether Dot felt it was important to keep the sentence about the cheerleader doll and basket of candy. Dot told me a story about Valley that caused me to conclude that, perhaps, Valley is the story.

Apparently, some folks loved Valley immediately, while others have grown to appreciate her. Absence does make the heart grow fonder, or so they say.

A couple of years ago, Dot noticed that Valley was missing from her perch in Dot's office. She searched but Valley was nowhere to be found. A couple of weeks later, Dot received an envelope with a rope tied around it. Inside was a note that read, "We have the doll. If you tell anyone in security, administration, or on the customer service team, the doll bites the dust." Dot decided it was time to take action. She circulated an e-mail that notified everyone of Valley's disappearance. Fearing for Valley's safety, she responsibly asked those expressly identified by the "doll-nappers" not to read the e-mail. The word was out. The hospital was abuzz with concern. Everyone began looking for Valley.

A couple of weeks later, Dot received an envelope that contained a photograph of Valley in front of Radio City Music Hall in New York City. A note from Valley's captor confirmed that Valley was safe and went on to relate how Valley coached her (the napper) to interact with a nasty taxi driver so that by the end of the ride, the cabby's attitude was quite pleasant. Not too long after that, a photograph of Valley surrounded by pelicans arrived—Valley was in Hawaii. Over a period of months, Dot received photographs showing Valley at the Grand Canyon, in Washington D.C., on the London Bridge, and dressed up for Halloween. Each photograph was delivered with a note from an accomplice, identifying how Valley was intervening to create positive customer experiences.

As mysteriously as she vanished, Valley eventually returned from her travels. Dot continues to make her "workout" rounds. And "she takes a cheerleader doll, appropriately named 'Valley,' and a basket filled with candy to share with all."

I loved this story because it is an amusing example of collaboration and team spirit and relates to a single reference to a doll—a reference I initially thought should come out of the profile because it diminished the significance of their achievements…little did I know.

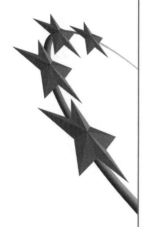

Huron Valley–
Sinai Hospital

Commerce, Mich.

Organizations that enjoy loyal customers are those whose customers consistently rate the service as "excellent," rather than simply "good." Providence Centralia Hospital introduced the SHAPE program to strengthen the satisfaction of patients, physicians, and employees. Continuous improvement and consistent service delivery enabled this community-based hospital to achieve impressive results.

Several factors pointed to the need for a strong customer service focus at Providence Centralia Hospital (PCH). These included weak patient and physician satisfaction scores, a general feeling of "unease" by our employees, and a worsening financial picture. A group of our leaders met to discuss how we could improve customer service. After identifying patients, physicians and co-workers as our three primary customer groups, we committed to improve the satisfaction of all three. We concluded that most of our customers experience good customer service on most days. However, we wanted to make sure that excellent service was delivered to all of our customers every day. The slogan we adopted, "Service Happens at Providence Everyday" and known by the acronym SHAPE, identified that commitment.

Forty-five members of the SHAPE Team, representing most departments of the hospital, met to discuss customer service and decided the focus should be on improving our interpersonal performance. Many activities highlighted our emphasis on improving interactions with our customers. These included placing posters around the hospital, publishing articles in the PCH newsletter, issuing customer service report cards to assess the impact of our efforts, holding staff meetings, rewarding SHAPE behaviors and having our administrator deliver numerous talks at staff meetings.

The following year, the SHAPE Team changed its focus to make SHAPE part of the PCH culture. We wanted to emphasize the importance of customer service from the time a potential employee interviews with PCH to the time that person leaves PCH. All managers and supervisors received sample questions to use during the interview process, which were designed to determine the applicant's knowledge of and commitment to customer service. Managers and supervisors began using a checklist of SHAPE topics to discuss during the interview process. New employees are asked to sign a commitment to live the core values of the Sisters of Providence Health System while at work.

SHAPE standards have been added to the annual performance appraisal. Patient care managers and supervisors have developed a system to meet with patients and make sure patients and families understand that they should expect to receive excellent customer service. Patients are encouraged to

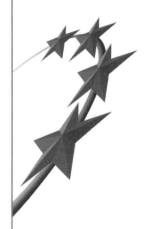

Providence
Centralia
Hospital

Centralia, Wash.

19

notify the manager or supervisor immediately if service does not meet that standard.

The next year, the SHAPE Team went even further. We knew we could not create satisfying experiences if systems prevented us from delivering excellent service. All departments identified a work process that acted as a barrier to providing excellent customer service. We wanted small, quick projects that could be finished within nine months. As a result, the lab improved its turnaround time for drug screen collections and breath alcohol determinations; CCU/ICU improved patient and family education on diabetes; surgery improved the orthopaedic charge process; diagnostic imaging improved report turnaround time; and rehab/TCU improved its discharge process.

In addition to improving patient satisfaction at PCH, we wanted to strengthen our relationships with physicians. To address this, we conducted interviews to identify how we could improve service to our physicians and their office staffs.

Within three years, our results looked much better. The percentage of patients who rated us as "excellent" went from 33% to 69%. The percentage of physicians who would "recommend PCH as a place to practice" went from 55% to 75%. Overall satisfaction experienced by employees went from 3.63 to 3.96 (on a scale of 5) and patient complaints related to employee attitude dropped from 33% to 13%. These improvements indicate that service happens at Providence Centralia every day!

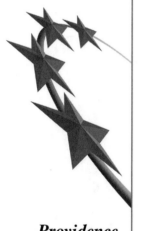

*Providence
Centralia
Hospital*

Centralia, Wash.

Whitman Hospital and Medical Center, a 32-bed acute care hospital serving the needs of a 12,000-square-mile area in Washington state, understands the importance of recognizing and rewarding excellent service. The initiatives Whitman has implemented have helped to build employee participation and patient satisfaction. Whitman celebrates in creative ways, which has contributed to improving its ranking to the 97th percentile among peer hospitals.

When Whitman Hospital and Medical Center began using a national firm to measure patient satisfaction, we began to hear success stories from other facilities and knew we needed to do more with regard to patient satisfaction. We formed a Care Team, made up of staff and managers and chaired by the director of performance improvement, to look at patient satisfaction issues. The Care Team was given a budget of $3,000 to use toward making improvements in patient satisfaction and internal customer service.

The Care Team decided to focus on improving the patient experience and developing a culture of excellence. As time went by, the team adopted the service theme, "WE CARE." This theme is also an acronym that stands for: Whitman, Employees, Customer-first, Attitude, Respect/Recover, and Excellence. A companion reward and recognition program was called "Caught Caring." Employees who are caught caring by other employees are recognized in the monthly employee newsletter and receive prizes, such as a free lunch, an extra half hour added to their lunch break, or being able to leave work a half hour early. A celebration is held to honor all those caught caring during the quarter, and these employees are entered into a drawing for a paid day off.

The team also identified some patient satisfaction issues that were easily dealt with. The team purchased long distance phone cards, coloring books, crayons, and other items that staff can give to patients or visitors, as appropriate. Employees received Customer Service Survival Kits, participated in customer service games, and watched educational videos. The Care Team announced that National Customer Service Week would be celebrated by focusing attention on "internal service" and the relationships we maintain with each other.

Another acronym, HAT, was adopted for our service recovery program: Hear the complaint; Apologize; Thank and take action. Staff can write personal notes and offer free lunch tickets, phone cards, items from the gift shop, or even cash, when they respond to complaints.

The team developed standards of behavior for employees. They are creating an admission brochure to welcome patients to our hospital, and promoting a "Shhh" campaign to reduce patients' complaints about noise.

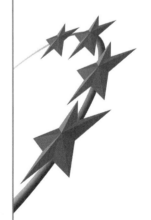

Whitman Hospital and Medical Center

Colfax, Wash.

In our custom peer group of small hospitals, our overall ranking went from the 85th to 93rd percentile within six months of launching our WE CARE initiative. The Care Team developed awards for excellence in patient satisfaction based on the survey results. The top award is called "Prize Winning Catch." It is a big pink fish named "Starfish" that is attached to an anchor. The anchor stays with the winning department and Starfish goes to the department that has the highest score on the next report. Another award is given to a support department that is not included on the patient satisfaction survey. It is called the "WHMC USS Lifesaver." The Care Team votes on the department to receive this award, which is a round life ring. "Hooked on Patient Satisfaction" certificates are given to departments and areas ranked in the 90th percentile or above.

To celebrate our success, we had a patient satisfaction celebration that all employees were invited to attend. The "Top Tuna," our CEO, dressed in an apron, rubber boots, and yellow rain cap, presented the above-mentioned awards. During the celebration, questions were asked regarding our patient satisfaction scores. Top Tuna tossed fish crackers and tuna cans out of his fishing creel to employees who gave correct answers. We also recognize departments that need to work on improvement with a prize called "The One That Got Away." This is a boat oar with a fish attached to it and it goes to the area that is ranked lowest on the report. The name of the item that was ranked lowest, such as "noise," is written on the fish to remind the department where attention must be focused. The fun we have with our awards and celebrations adds to the spirit of our organization and the ways WE CARE.

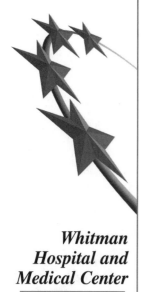

Whitman Hospital and Medical Center

Colfax, Wash.

Resident satisfaction was below the national mean and over half the employee workforce had departed for greener landscapes overlooking the Susquehanna River. Within 24 months of when Ideal Senior Living Center introduced its Red Carpet℠ program, satisfaction improved from the 18th to the 92nd percentile at the skilled-nursing center and from the 14th to the 99th percentile in the independent living section. Just as impressive was the effect on employee turnover, which went from 54% to 23%.

The inspiration for our Red Carpet℠ program came when the CEO of Ideal Senior Living Center was on vacation and placed an order in a restaurant. The CEO responded to a waiter's inquiry about salad dressing by saying, "I don't want salad dressing…and please, no tomatoes, no onions…just mozzarella cheese and croutons." The typical response to this is, "I'll check, but there may not be any mozzarella cheese…" or "I'm sorry, it's already prepared in the kitchen." This waiter—without a moment of hesitation—said, "When you're a guest in my house, you can have anything you want."

That single phrase eventually had a transformational effect on Ideal Senior Living's service culture. The CEO returned to work convinced that residents deserve to feel "wowed" by the same attitude. After sharing her story, members of the management team began sharing their own similar experiences in hotels, restaurants, veterinarians' offices, etc., which resulted in the feeling they received "red carpet treatment." Not too long afterward, Ideal rolled out our Red Carpet℠ program.

The Red Carpet℠ program began with first impressions. Each entrance soon bore a sign announcing "Ideal rolls out the RED CARPET for YOU." We placed red carpets at every entrance. Warm greetings are extended by employees when visitors arrive. Guests are asked if they would like to be escorted to their destinations.

Managers and supervisors received intensive training to learn what must be done to "wow" customers. Key phrases for the program were coined, such as "Welcome to Ideal" and "Have an Ideal Day." Before leaving the resident, staff says, "Is there anything else I can do before I leave?" All residents receive a welcome letter and personal visit from the President/CEO, as well as visits from key managers.

Since families are an integral part of our residents' lives, managers attend family meetings and other functions on a routine basis. Managers mingle, asking families and residents how they would rate the services and inquiring about what improvements are necessary to achieve their utmost satisfaction. If dissatisfaction exists, issues can be addressed promptly.

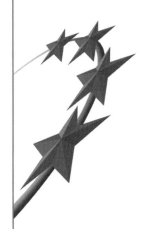

Ideal Senior Living Center
Endicott, N.Y.

Group meetings are held with families and residents, asking them to rate each department and identify any areas or opportunities for improvement. With the Red Carpet℠ program, communication is key.

Employees participated on teams and developed standards of behavior, reward and recognition programs, and ways to recover from mishaps. It was critical that senior and middle management be visible and "walk the talk." Managers began making rounds routinely to ensure that employees had the training and supplies necessary to perform their jobs.

From our research, we also learned that if our employees were satisfied, our residents would be satisfied. We developed a Red Carpet℠ program for employees. Using service maps, we created an "awesome arrival" for applicants and new hires. The job application form and process were redesigned. Every applicant is greeted by a member of the human resource team and offered an on-the-spot interview, if they prefer. When they leave, they are always given a date when they will be informed about the hiring decision. Once hired, they receive a welcome note from the president/CEO within 24 hours, a call from their supervisor within 48 hours, and subsequent calls from various individuals at Ideal welcoming them to the team.

We now practice the philosophy that recruitment is not the job of human resources, but every manager's responsibility. Employees are invited to lunch with the president at a local restaurant to celebrate one month, one year, and subsequent annual anniversaries. Once a month, the President/CEO hosts a "Getting to Know You" reception at which coffee and pastries are served in the lobby during all three shifts.

A revelation for Ideal was learning the value of analyzing and interpreting data from our satisfaction surveys. In the past, we received results, moaned and groaned about not reaching the mean, and then hoped to do better. Now, we identify the top three or four indicators that drive satisfaction, create action plans to improve performance, and act on them. Employees take responsibility for results, as well. They understand the impact their attitudes and actions have on resident and family satisfaction.

Friendliness and cheerfulness surround us at Ideal. In 12 months, our ranking in overall satisfaction went from the 18th to the 88th percentile at the skilled nursing center, from the 7th to the 80th percentile in our independent living area, and from the 14th to the 87th percentile in our assisted living area. Twelve months following, all units consistently maintain strong performance in the >90th percentile. Our employee turnover has gone from 54.8% to 23.2%. Ideal is proud of our success with the Red Carpet℠ program. We will continue to "roll out the red carpet" and welcome success in the future.

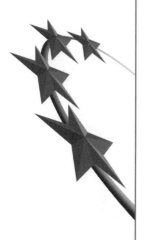

Ideal Senior Living Center

Endicott, N.Y.

When Yakima Valley Memorial Hospital was offered the opportunity to purchase an extended care facility, leaders realized the acquisition would help resolve the problem of providing convalescent care to patients who no longer qualified to stay in the acute care hospital. This also gave the hospital the chance to realize its vision of creating "a continuum of comfort-driven, high-quality health care." A planning team worked to transform a nursing home that was sorely in need of both facility and program renovations into a place of comfort and hope for patients. This vision resulted in a dynamic healing environment called, Garden Village.

Yakima Valley Memorial Hospital (YVMH) is located in the center of the state of Washington. The region it serves is one of the poorest in the state. Consequently, the hospital has one of the largest Medicaid and Medicare patient loads in the region. Amounts allocated to charity care continue to climb every year.

Two issues facing health care in America—reimbursement rates that do not fully cover the cost of care and limitations on patient hospital stays—pose a multitude of challenges to acute-care facilities. Perhaps the greatest challenge is to figure out how to provide a continuum of comfort-driven, high-quality health care despite the obstacles.

Our primary dilemma was how to provide continuing care for convalescing patients whose health care plans determined that further hospitalization was too expensive. These patients, often young and with full presence of mind, faced continued recuperation at home without benefits of needed therapies or nursing support. The alternative was to receive rehabilitation services and nursing care in a traditional nursing home setting.

When the owner of a group of nursing homes offered to sell one of the properties, Central Convalescent Center, we recognized the opportunity to extend high-quality health care beyond the hospital walls "Memorial-style." By purchasing this facility, we had the potential to attain our vision of providing a healing environment where mind, body, and spirit are addressed by merging clinical care with hotel-style hospitality.

The newly acquired facility was renamed Garden Village. Its employees immediately began benefiting from the opportunity to work with Memorial employees who specialized in surgical recovery and orthopaedic care, as well as respiratory, occupational, and physical therapy. Today, these hospital departments work directly with Garden Village staff to coordinate procedures and standards of care between the hospital and long term care facility for both short term patients recovering from recent hospitalization and patients who will spend the rest of their lives in long term care.

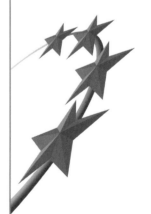

Yakima Valley Memorial Hospital

Yakima, Wash.

"Hotel-style hospitality" arrived via the two support departments brought in to assist with the transformation of Garden Village: YVMH's general services and food service departments. Both managers began their assessment of the facility with thorough on-site inspections and interviews of supervisors, staff members, patients, and patient family members. Managers discovered that, in addition to equipment needs, staff morale was low and basic quality and customer service practices required upgrading.

Garden Village identified nine key areas for improving the facility's housekeeping and laundry services: 1) adopting higher standards, 2) adjusting labor, 3) restructuring shifts and staffing, 4) naming a single coordinator for several departments, 5) defining better job descriptions, 6) improving relationships with patient care staff, 7) offering hospitality and customer service training, 8) improving standard equipment and uniforms, and 9) improving the existing quality assurance program.

Specific actions were identified to improve all of these areas. The assessment revealed food service practices were below the hospital's high standards, and that patients had few choices at mealtime. Patients and family members communicated that they wanted food service to be more like that of YVMH. Garden Village's menu was redesigned to offer gourmet main courses and specialty desserts. Customer service practices were modified to include personal visits by the food service staff each week to educate and help patients select menu items.

As these programmatic changes took place, Garden Village underwent a physical transformation. Faded and stained rooms received hardwood floors, fresh paint, and natural-toned textured wall treatments. Interior appointments, plants, and live birds were added to make patients feel more at home. Common areas where patients could gather and get away from their rooms were created. New, beautifully landscaped garden and patio areas created new spaces for patient enjoyment. In addition, special rooms and beds were set aside for orthopaedic hospital patients in need of follow-up convalescent care. When the physical renovations were completed, Garden Village was fully transformed and this beautiful facility was made an independent, stand-alone, not-for-profit entity.

Before improvements were initiated, Central Convalescent Center maintained an average patient census of 79%. Today, the average census at Garden Village is 92%. A recent patient and family survey indicated 96% satisfaction in areas related to staff, food, and facility cleanliness. The survey feedback is consistent with satisfaction expressed by members of the Patient Concern Committee and the resident and family councils. Their satisfaction recognizes the contributions made by members of the Garden Village team, without which we could not have achieved our vision and success.

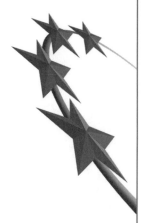

Yakima Valley Memorial Hospital

Yakima, Wash.

The Planetree model of patient-centered care is focused on personalizing, humanizing and demystifying patients' and families' health care experiences. Griffin Hospital embarked on a culture-changing transformation to become patient-centered and service-driven when it opened the first patient care building in the country designed as a healing environment based on the Planetree Model. Since that time, it has experienced phenomenal growth in patient admissions and outpatient services, superb patient satisfaction ratings, and widespread recognition as being a provider of quality care in the community and a progressive leader in the industry. Earning a distinction that is rarely extended to health care organizations, Griffin Hospital has been named by Fortune magazine as one of the "100 Best Companies to Work for in America" for five consecutive years.

Griffin Hospital is committed to deliver personalized, humanistic care in a healing environment that results in unique care experiences for patients and families. With the completion of a $30 million facilities improvement program, we opened a new patient care building in 1994. This new facility was designed to complement the Planetree philosophy of patient-centered care.

Griffin's facility provides a hotel-like environment. Each patient unit has a kitchen that can be used by patients and family members, and where volunteers regularly bake cookies, muffins and other treats for customers. There are quiet lounges with salt-water aquariums and entertainment lounges with pianos. Patient units are carpeted. Soft colors, wood treatments, indirect lighting, and beautiful artwork are used extensively to create a soothing environment.

Instead of one central nursing station, there are decentralized nursing stations for every four beds. A primary care nurse is assigned to each of these stations, providing greater proximity and accessibility to/for patients and their families. Each unit has a health library that contains educational materials including books, videos, and audio tapes, as well as Internet access for patient and family use. Patients and visitors are welcomed with music in parking lots. Concierge-like volunteers, who are members of our Ambassador program, greet patients and visitors in the lobby. Patients have access to 64 television channels including a meditation channel and an education channel. We do not charge for television, parking, or telephone services.

The Planetree model includes unrestricted, around-the-clock visitation throughout the hospital, including the critical care unit. Patients have access to their medical records, in which they may write their own comments. Massages are given by trained volunteers; entertainment is offered by musicians, magicians, caricaturists; meal service is delivered hotel-style;

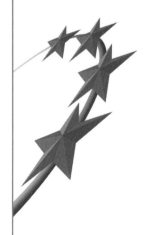

Griffin Hospital

Derby, Conn.

and a pet therapy program that includes 22 specially-trained and certified dogs is available.

Patients are expected to become partners in their treatment and care. Within 24 hours of admission, patients receive a packet of information about their medical condition that includes recent medical research. A patient care conference, held within 48 hours of admission, includes the patient and family members, primary care nurse, attending physicians and social work staff. Patient Pathways that describe, in lay terms, the day-by-day plan for care, tests, and procedures are distributed to patients and family members.

Griffin recently completed hospital-wide integration of the Planetree philosophy by expanding the model to our 14-bed inpatient psychiatric unit. The unit incorporates Planetree's healing design principles, including the elimination of barriers between patients and staff. Comfortable public spaces encourage social interaction and the involvement of family. The combination of design and technology protects patient privacy and enhances patient and staff safety.

A Community Health Resource Center (CHRC) is adjacent to the main entrance. The CHRC is a lending library and houses one of the largest collections of lay, professional health and medical publications in the country, as well as an extensive collection of audio and videotapes. The center provides Internet access to users, and staff is trained to assist patients in researching medical information. Over 25,000 users access the services of the center every year, including over 9,000 residents of the community who have CHRC lending cards.

Our commitment to education extends to employees. A two-day, overnight, off-site retreat is conducted at an austere convent to help employees see the hospital experience through the patient's eyes. Employees stay in simple rooms with bunk beds and no private bathrooms, televisions or telephones. The one entrée served at mealtime is whatever the nuns are eating. Participants are asked to feed each other to demonstrate how disenabling the hospital experience can be. Every employee is considered a caregiver and to date about 1,000 employees have attended the retreats. A full-day new employee orientation is presented by members of the executive team and focuses on organizational values, culture, and service excellence.

"I Take It Personally" is the identity of an employee recognition program that provides $250 awards every month to four employees who demonstrate exceptional patient service. The employee of the year receives a $1,000 award. "Success rewards" are paid quarterly to associates and individual department members for achieving specific targets related to patient satisfaction, business growth, and productivity.

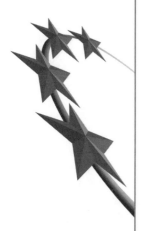

Griffin Hospital

Derby, Conn.

Our ultimate success is measured by patient satisfaction and the community's perception of the quality and care at Griffin Hospital. We contract with a market research company to conduct monthly telephone surveys and use what is referred to as a Secured Customer Rating (SCR) to measure success. To become a secured customer, the patient must give Griffin the highest possible rating on two dimensions—willingness to return and willingness to recommend. Griffin's SCR was 82% for the current fiscal year. Overall patient satisfaction averages 98%. The same monthly survey is done for 100 emergency department patients. The SCR in the ED is 70% and the patient satisfaction rating is 94%.

The same company also does a biannual community telephone survey of 360 primary and 200 secondary service area residents, all randomly selected. In the most recent survey, residents rated Griffin the most improved hospital of eight hospitals in the region by a 3-to-1 margin, and quality of care higher than other area hospitals. Griffin also uses quarterly mailed surveys to measure patient satisfaction with outpatient services. Each outpatient department has specific patient satisfaction targets that are part of their goals and on which success rewards are paid. In the latest survey, eight of nine departments exceeded their satisfaction targets, and the average for all departments was over 95%.

Our unique facility, care model, and commitment to service excellence are making Griffin the hospital of choice for employees, as well as consumers. For five consecutive years, Griffin has been named by Fortune magazine as one of the "100 Best Companies to Work for in America." We currently rank 26th on that list. Griffin is one of the fastest growing and most profitable hospitals in Connecticut. Our patient admissions increased nearly 28% over a three-year period, compared with growth rates of 6-8% for other hospitals. Use of outpatient services is up more than 60% over four years. Solucient named Griffin one of the nation's top performance improvement leaders based on five years of quality, operating, and financial data.

The Planetree philosophy at Griffin Hospital is responsive to the changing expectations of patients, the growing needs of our community, the dynamic forces that impact the industry's performance, and the discerning expectations of employees.

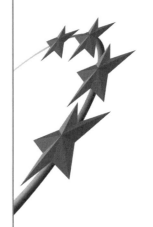

Griffin
Hospital

Derby, Conn.

Despite its longstanding popularity in Europe, the practice of giving women the option of water births is a more recent emerging trend in America. At a time in history when women are going "retro" and asking for epidurals to relieve pain in childbirth, North Shore Birth Center, a freestanding birthing center on the grounds of Beverly Hospital, is committed to gentle birthing and to give women in the community the choice of water births in or outside of the hospital setting. Loyal customers emerge from the alternative birthing experience.

The mission of "giving childbirth back to women" is embraced by the North Shore Birth Center. Midwives, traditionally, have incorporated the use of warm water while a mother is in labor, using hot water bottles, warm showers, baths, and compresses to relieve the discomfort of contractions. Women often enjoy the comfort a warm bath provides during labor because it induces relaxation and decreases anxiety; stepping out of a tub to deliver the baby can be a jarring interruption.

Immersion in water during birth, as well as during labor, has been used in Europe for many years. The first birthing pool was installed in a hospital in Great Britain in 1987. By 1993, all maternity units in England and Wales had managed labor or delivery in water, and nearly half had installed birthing pools. Popularity of water births has increased in the U.S. over the years but adoption of the practice has not been as pronounced as in Europe.

The notion of water births in this country has become appealing to many women. Women search for practices that will accommodate their desires. Our offer of water births is in response to patients' preferences and requests. Prior to its inception at North Shore Birth Center, our staff did extensive research. We hired a midwife with experience attending water births to give an in-service to our staff. Some of our physicians were reluctant at first, but they approved our new protocol and agreed to support us in our new undertaking. We purchased a portable Aqua Doula® tub and began soon after. We have recently joined a Web site that lists facilities offering water births. Our own Web site includes this information. Word of mouth has also directed patients our way.

For those patients who have successfully delivered their babies in the tub, we have received nothing but rave reviews resulting from patients' comfort, satisfaction, and gratitude for providing this service.

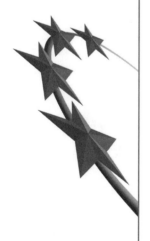

**North Shore
Birth Center**

Beverly, Mass.

Women are key health care consumers. Designing health care services for this important segment of the market requires a unique understanding of women's preferences and an awareness of changing trends. Before breaking ground to build a new specialty hospital for women and babies, Lancaster General Hospital involved physicians, nurses, other professionals, and community members in the planning. Their involvement provided assurance that the new hospital would reflect the desires of women in the community, and fill unmet needs.

Maternity services are only the beginning at Lancaster General Women & Babies Hospital. Not only do we deliver more babies than any other hospital in Lancaster County, we also provide comprehensive women's health services including diagnostic testing, breast care, osteoporosis diagnosis and prevention, menopause education and counseling, fitness and wellness programs, and inpatient and outpatient surgery. Lancaster General provides services that are customized to fit women's needs at every stage of life.

Members of our community, medical staff, hospital board of directors, nurses, administrators, and other allied health professionals collaborated on the plans that would enable Lancaster General Hospital to achieve its vision to provide health care services for women and their families. Team members had the clinical expertise and knowledge of patient needs. These individuals were also well aware of trends in the health care industry and the types of technologies and services that are needed to be state-of-the-art. We invited community members to share their input because they represented their fellow county residents and spoke to what women and men would like to see. These individuals were divided into five work teams, including clinical patient services, operations/systems, financial, facility, and community relations/marketing. These teams helped turn our vision into a functional hospital.

Specific to the needs of maternity patients, we identified guiding principles that included four objectives:

- The environment created will be family-centered and provide a celebratory birthing experience.

- Patient choice will be prioritized and patients will actively control health care decisions and services.

- The facility will serve the unique health care and preventive needs of women and their families.

- The facility will offer services and amenities as desired by women and their families.

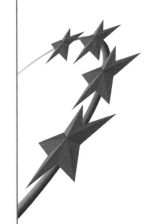

Lancaster General Women & Babies Hospital

Lancaster, Pa.

From our conversations and studies, we established several requirements for maternity patients at our new women's hospital: 1) open visitation; 2) a separate labor and delivery area (not an LDRP model); 3) private rooms with private baths and Jacuzzi tubs; 4) a large family waiting room with kitchenette; 5) ten on-call rooms for physicians and midwives; 6) two nurseries and four operating rooms; 7) a café, gift shop, and spacious lobby for visitors; 8) outpatient women's services, including mammography and laboratory testing; 9) restaurant-style meals and a complimentary meal for the father: and 10) immediate access to anesthesia and other pain relief options for laboring mothers.

Even now, we continue to make modifications when we identify performance improvement opportunities. We have a dedicated process improvement team for the hospital. This team reports to Performance Improvement Council at Lancaster General Hospital and has successfully implemented various multidisciplinary process changes. This committee monitors the effectiveness of changes to ensure they are having the desired result.

A noteworthy example of process improvement in action involves our plans for a new special care unit. We identified the need for a higher level of care to accommodate high-risk OB patients and to care for more complicated cases after birth. This will allow us to keep mother and baby together and avoid transferring the mother to our main hospital. Other improvements have included: 1) anesthesia/surgery post-cesarean birth orders that delineate the responsible party for pain management during each stage of recovery following cesarean births, 2) 48-hour post-discharge follow-up phone calls, and 3) pre-anesthesia screening of 100% of our patients to identify individuals with risk factors and co-morbid conditions prior to delivery.

Since opening, we have witnessed a significant increase in patient volumes and patient satisfaction. Through verbal and written comments and surveys, patients and their families have shared their appreciation for the services we provide. Our markct share has increased from 49% to 60% in our first year and to 65% in our second year. The first three months of the current fiscal year indicate a 16% increase in patient volumes, which should significantly impact our market share. We achieved an operating margin of $2.4 million at the end of the first year; a projected loss of over $2 million had been budgeted.

Our new hospital's patient satisfaction scores reflect our instant success. The hospital's overall satisfaction score increased by five percentage points in three months. The "likelihood of recommending to friends and family" score increased by 6 points and has continued to increase to a high of 96.1. Our current patient satisfaction score is 89.3. This is 6.5 points higher than scores reported by hospitals in our benchmark database and puts us in the top 1% in customer satisfaction among hospitals surveyed by our vendor.

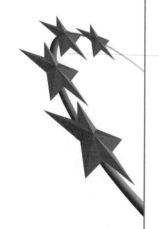

Lancaster General
Women & Babies
Hospital

Lancaster, Pa.

Some 68% of patients rated us as "very good" in our first year. All of this was accomplished while serving an ever-increasing number of customers. In the first year, our volumes increased 22%; second year volumes increased 7%. Although we are meeting the needs of our inpatient population, we realize that we must continually strive to meet all of the needs of women and families in our community.

We have added several new perinatology services, antepartum testing, hearing screening for newborns, and a postpartum depression program that helps patients and their loved ones identify the early signs of postpartum depression and treatment options. Lancaster General Women & Babies Hospital also offers a comprehensive, multidisciplinary approach to diseases of the breast at its Breast Care Center. The Women's Health Boutique provides prosthetics, wigs, compression devices, incontinence supplies, and other items for women. We developed a menopause program to help women recognize the short term discomforts and meet the challenges of menopause. The Women's Resource and Wellness Center is also situated on the campus to provide educational materials and access to Internet research.

Our facility is smaller than a community acute care facility and it creates a feeling of intimacy. Our staff knows each other by name and works cohesively as a team. Because of this, everyone who enters the hospital senses the warmth and friendliness evident throughout the facility, from the greeters to the security guards, nurses, and physicians.

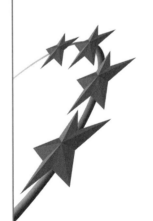

Lancaster General
Women & Babies
Hospital

Lancaster, Pa.

The obstetrics unit at Columbia Memorial Hospital had remained essentially the same for 40 years, in a time warp bypassed by the revolution in childbirth practices that occurred over the past two decades. As a result, increasing numbers of patients chose to go elsewhere to have their babies. When the time came to renovate the unit and adopt a family-centered care model, the hospital involved unit staff, physicians, and representatives from other key departments in the planning. This helped to assure that the facility, as well as the care delivered at the Family Birth Place, would respond to patient needs and preferences. It also served to respond to the staff needs and preferences. After extensive renovations and reorientation of staff, 88% of patients were very satisfied with the care provided, compared with 60% who were very satisfied in previous years.

The obstetrics unit renovation and work redesign project was the first in a series of projects generated by Columbia Memorial Hospital's (CMH) master plan. The vision for the new Family Birth Place was that every woman would have the opportunity to give birth as she wishes, in an environment where she felt nurtured and secure, and where her emotional well-being, privacy, and personal preferences were respected. To achieve that, it was essential that we view this project through the eyes of those who deliver care to patients.

Maternity staff, obstetricians, nurse-midwives, pediatricians, family practitioners, and anesthesia staff worked with architects, engineering, and bio-medical departments to design a birthing unit that would incorporate high-tech equipment in a comfortable home-like setting for patients. These groups held bi-weekly meetings for more than 18 months as renovations were planned. The nursing staff drove many of the decisions for this unit. Staff visited other facilities to view layouts, furnishings and to speak with peers about construction considerations, operational efficiencies, and patient care conveniences. Most meetings with architects were held on the obstetrics unit so all staff could give input. Each generation of the plan was posted in the lounge for further discussion. To show their approval, each member of the OB staff and key departments that participated in the planning were asked to sign the final plans. Prior to signing this agreement, nurses communicated their concerns that the nursery was not fully visible from the nursing station. Our board of trustees respected the staff's judgment and concerns about security and agreed to a significant increase in the project budget to remedy the situation.

Nine to 12 months prior to completion of the renovations, we initiated a work redesign project. Our unit's staffing is comprised of 92% RNs and the goal is not only to maintain this complement but to assure that each nurse is competent and cross-trained to provide labor, delivery, postpartum, and

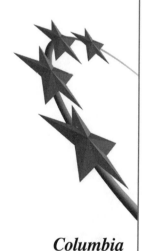

*Columbia
Memorial
Hospital*

Hudson, N.Y.

newborn care. This patient care delivery model allows for the same nurse to care for the mother from the time of admission until discharge. The patient is admitted to one room and remains in this room throughout her stay. The newborn also rooms with the mother, except when moms request additional time for rest. The redesign provides for fewer patient moves, more privacy, better continuity of care, and permits new fathers to stay overnight with mom and baby. It also allows the same nursing staff to teach, support, and transition the patient to the role of new mother.

The plan was carefully thought out to provide maximum flexibility so that multiple functions and unusual peaks in census could be accommodated without building expensive, unneeded space. A cluster of pre-existing labor rooms was repainted and is now used as call rooms for staff. They can be pressed into use if more labor rooms are needed. A large family lounge is used for education including prenatal and breastfeeding instruction, sibling classes, and safe-sitter classes.

Each discharged patient is mailed a satisfaction survey. Scores continue to rank the care provided at the 90th percentile or better. Complimentary letters are received by the nursing staff, administration and trustees on a regular basis. One example of a complimentary letter from a new parent stated, "You taught us that birth is a team effort and we learned childbirth isn't something to be feared, but a time to work together to bring forth joy that nothing else can match. We only wish that all families could know childbirth as it was meant to be."

We continue to market our new service. Education efforts have improved to include a certified RN lactation consultant because of the increase in breastfeeding among new mothers. CMH has recruited three new OB/GYN practitioners to our hospital where they can practice in a flexible, modern environment with state-of-the-art equipment and clinically competent staff.

Every member of our staff with OB privileges is certified in neonatal resuscitation. CMH is one of nine hospitals in New York state to achieve this level of certification and received the "Special Delivery Award" by the American Academy of Pediatrics. Anesthesia, nursing, and medical staff designed options for analgesia during labor that were not previously available. A hydrotherapy tub in a garden-like room complete with soft music, lighting and aromatherapy, facilitates relaxation during labor. A family kitchen and playroom for children are available to the mother, her family and support team. All registered nurses have been trained in labor management, delivery, postpartum care and newborn care.

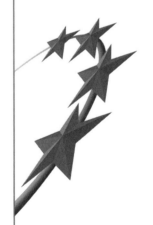

Columbia Memorial Hospital

Hudson, N.Y.

Our patient satisfaction scores have improved and deliveries have increased since the project was completed. One year after the opening of the Family Birth Place, a CMH study of local households utilizing our OB services revealed 88% were very satisfied with care provided in the last year, compared with 60% being very satisfied in the last five years. Prior to our change in the delivery of care, survey results demonstrated 93% of patients rated our OB service very good or excellent. OB volume has increased from 474 births before the center, to 510 the next year. Payor mix has shifted by 10% from Medicaid to commercial payors, indicating patients of a higher socio-economic level are choosing our facility for their birth experience. The average tenure of staff working on this unit is 14 years, pointing to employee satisfaction with the workplace environment.

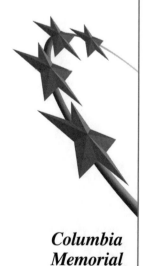

*Columbia
Memorial
Hospital*

Hudson, N.Y.

CHAPTER 2
TEAM INITIATIVES

TEAM INITIATIVES

Soon after Beaumont Hospital–Troy unveiled its vision to be a hospital driven by customer satisfaction, the ambition to "strive for fives" was unleashed. Inpatient satisfaction ascended throughout the hospital, but the obstetrics unit found it difficult to achieve similar outcomes and decided to find out why. Not only did overall patient satisfaction improve as a result of their initiatives, but the staff learned how to better respond to patients' spiritual needs and to reduce noise and disruption on the unit.

At Beaumont Hospital–Troy, we began to notice that as the number of births and our market share increased, the satisfaction of our patients decreased. In an effort to accommodate the growing number of obstetrical (OB) patients, we had extended our main unit and were using beds located on a separate unit to accommodate overflow. The hospital's Inpatient Best Practice Committee partnered with us to analyze the impact this was having on patient satisfaction. We compared the satisfaction of patients by location and discovered significant differences. Although the scores for our main unit, with private rooms, were only at the 58th percentile, the scores for the overflow unit with semi-private rooms were in the 5th percentile. Neither was acceptable. We had to react quickly to improve customer satisfaction or risk losing market share.

We began making rounds to interact with our patients more frequently and learn how we could better respond to patient needs. We developed scripts so the information we provided and the ways we responded would be more consistent. We also decided that once a patient was placed on the main unit, she could not be transferred to the overflow unit. We developed service recovery procedures to remedy dissatisfaction.

Meanwhile, the hospital planned for a larger OB unit in a new addition that was being built on the campus. All rooms on the new unit would be private, with wider benches in the rooms for visitor comfort. Galleys would allow family members to get something to eat, and storage closets, accessible from the outer hall, would help to decrease patient disturbances. Although we realized the new physical space would help to improve patient satisfaction, we were conscious not to view the new unit as the answer to all our problems. We focused on two areas of concern that were listed in the top 10 of our priority index: 1) the degree to which staff addressed the emotional/spiritual needs of the patient, and 2) the noise level in and around the room.

The issue of addressing patients' emotional and spiritual needs had been discussed frequently. This area constantly appeared among the top five in our priority index so we pulled surveys that rated this dimension less than a five and called approximately 100 patients to gain better insight into why

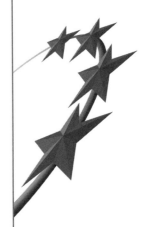

Beaumont Hospital–Troy

Troy, Mich.

they rated it the way they did. Once we had collected the feedback, we determined that we needed to be more proactive in letting patients know of our interest in supporting them emotionally or spiritually while they were hospitalized. Cards that invite patients to express any needs they may have in this regard are now distributed. Nurses are instructed to contact staff in social work or pastoral care when interest is expressed by patients. Simply taking the time to address this potential need with the patients helps to alleviate feelings that we do not care about what may be important to them. This solution helped to produce an increase in that particular score from 78.2 (20th percentile) to 84.9 (86th percentile). As a result, these cards are now used throughout the hospital.

Another one of our low ranking scores was in response to the question about the noise level in and around the patient rooms. Our mean score was 70.9, which placed us in the 28th percentile. An informal telephone poll was conducted and patients were asked about the noises that were most bothersome. We discovered that although patients did find noise coming from nursing stations to be bothersome, they reported that other patients and visitors also contributed noise that interfered with their rest and recuperation.

The committee created a poster campaign to remind everyone to be quiet and respectful. The posters featured children saying, "Shhh!" Employees were invited to bring their children, ages three to seven years, to an all-day photo session that was held on a Saturday. They were instructed to dress their child in clothing that represented something significant to the child. Approximately 50 children were photographed saying, "Shhh!" A poster was created of each child, all of which are displayed around the OB unit.

After hanging the posters, we noticed that the scores related to noise disturbance began to climb. The latest OB satisfaction scores for this dimension rank us in the 77th percentile. Because of the positive impact this campaign has had, the posters are now being utilized throughout the hospital.

These two improvements helped to improve the performance of our unit in meeting the needs and exceeding the expectations of our patients. Our overall satisfaction scores rose to the 95th percentile within six months. We now provide a happy, restful, and respectful environment for parents to bring children into the world.

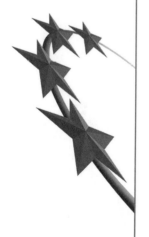

Beaumont Hospital–Troy

Troy, Mich.

By focusing on one service standard a month and introducing fun activities to remind staff of the service behaviors that contribute to patient satisfaction, the orthopedic unit at Concord Hospital succeeded in improving patient satisfaction. They assembled a Patient & Staff Satisfaction Team, known by the acronym P-S-S-T, and used various tools such as newsletters and contests to educate and motivate unit staff.

Wearing a blindfold, someone attempts to pour a glass of water. Another has donned a patient gown and a third person is wearing earplugs. These are examples of what you might find at Concord Hospital's P-S-S-T Meetings. What is P-S-S-T? And why would we do such things?

With inpatient survey scores repeatedly ranking in the 92nd to 96th percentile range, one might think there is little need to improve patient satisfaction at Concord Hospital. But even though the hospital's overall scores were high, the orthopedic unit's scores indicated there was room for improvement. It was time to take action. The unit's director formed a team of enthusiastic staff willing to commit the time and energy to learn how to become more customer-focused while working with patients, families, and other staff members. Employees from all shifts came together, including nurses, nurses' aides, housekeepers, and secretaries, as well as representatives from the spiritual care and quality assurance departments. Team members would, in turn, show others on the unit how to master the skills.

At the kick-off meeting, the director and the team's co-leaders served lunch to the new team members. Each person received a candle with a key tied to it, as a reminder that they were lighting the way and that each held the key to patient satisfaction. The team chose the name "P-S-S-T" or Patient & Staff Satisfaction Team, and adopted the motto, *"Psst! ... Have you heard? We've got a lot to do!"*

The team adopted a red flower and rainbow as its symbols after hearing Harry Chapin's song, *"Flowers Are Red."* These symbols are reminders that things don't have to remain the same because all flowers are not red; and it's OK to try new ideas to see all the colors in the rainbow. Team members wear buttons with these symbols and posters, banners, and other publications display them.

Service behaviors became our focus. Each month, one service behavior is selected. On randomly selected days and shifts, the hospital's president and chief executive officer, chief operating officer or chief nursing officer take turns performing "Goodie Rounds." Unit staff members are offered snacks if they know the behavior of the month. These rounds provide opportunities for management and staff to discuss how the current behavior is evidenced, and also demonstrate the level of commitment to customer satisfaction that is extended at Concord Hospital.

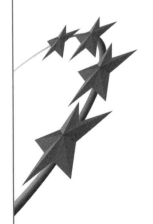

Concord Hospital

Concord, N.H.

One of the behaviors was "Keep It Quiet" and the value of this reinforcement approach was evident when the most recent patient satisfaction report indicated an improvement of 3.2 points on the survey dimension relating to noise. Staff members have made a conscious effort to keep noise levels down by using "nighttime" voices, shutting doors of patient rooms when appropriate, and doing the report at the time of shift changes in a conference room located away from patient areas. Staff found other opportunities to reduce noise such as setting pagers to "vibrate," moving a printer that was near a patient room, and fixing a door that constantly slammed.

A behavior is featured each month. Staff members "caught in the act" of performing the current month's service behavior are entered into a contest. The winner and the person who submitted the nomination are awarded certificates that can be redeemed in either the hospital cafeteria or ice cream stand. All nominations are published in the P-S-S-T newsletter distributed monthly on the orthopedic unit. The newsletter includes news of interest about people on the unit, customer service suggestions, and positive feedback from patients. These comments from our patients are also featured on posters that are displayed around the unit for all staff, patients, and visitors to see.

The orthopedic unit's "overall rating of care" jumped from 88.9 to 91.8 in the seven months since the team began. *Psst! ... have you heard?* Our score for that survey question now ranks us in the 96th percentile among hospitals.

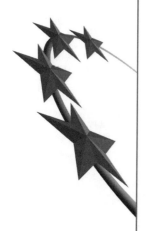

***Concord
Hospital***

Concord, N.H.

When The St. Luke Hospital West rededicated its efforts to achieve high levels of patient satisfaction, the emphasis was on every department's contribution, and managers were held accountable for results. The transitional care unit had consistently received low scores. The manager of the unit accepted responsibility to change this persistent outcome. In the space of a few months, the unit experienced a dramatic turnaround, going from the lowest to the highest scoring unit in the hospital.

The St. Luke Hospital West adopted the motto, "PRIDE in our Service to You," when it launched the customer service program. But the patient satisfaction scores for the transitional care unit (TCU) did not make us proud. During a three month period, our score dropped to 78.9%, which was the lowest ever reported and lower than any other unit in the hospital.

This was unacceptable to the staff on the unit, as well as to senior leaders of the hospital. In a meeting with the senior vice president, the unit manager was informed that the satisfaction scores were her responsibility to improve.

At the first staff meeting, the manager outlined what customer service meant to her, as well as to the unit, hospital, and staff. The manager was enthusiastic and projected her enthusiasm. Together the unit team members formulated a goal and direction. The goal was for the TCU to be the friendliest unit any of our patients had ever experienced or even imagined.

The next day, the manager began making daily patient rounds, visiting every patient and immediately addressing any issues that were identified. The manager became the role model and took staff members into rooms with her to discuss patient concerns. The manager wanted the staff to understand that patients' goals, wishes, and priorities did not necessarily match medical and nursing priorities. The lesson was that the patient care team must invest extra effort to discern the human, emotional needs of patients and to meet these whenever possible.

The first rule was developed: At the beginning of each shift, find out what is important for each patient that day and strive to meet that need. A second rule was adopted: Every time you enter a patient's room, make sure all the patient's current needs are met before leaving. This led to a third rule: Avoid setting yourself up for failure. The teaching point developed from this advice was to predict how long something would take but to be realistic when setting an expectation, then to exceed the prediction.

After a few weeks, the staff began rounding in the same manner. The manager then assumed the role of a resource provider. Staff members called the manager when they needed help meeting special needs, such as helping a patient's wife get some things from a store. Another patient's most ardent wish was to receive a visit from her dog. Could we do it? We did!

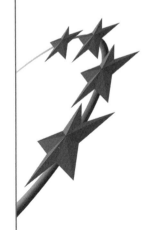

The St. Luke Hospital West

Florence, Ky.

The next quarter's score was up to 81.4, and the unit celebrated. Trend graphs were posted with messages saying *"great job"* or *"way to go."* Questionnaires returned with comments were used to show the staff how well they were doing. A poster was made of all the names of staff mentioned in the survey questionnaires, which spurred healthy competition throughout the unit to see who could get mentioned the most times.

Scores continued to rise to 83.1 in the next quarter, then to 83.9 in the following quarter. As scores rose, nurses and other staff members saw their names mentioned more frequently. Something else wonderful happened… the employees became happier with their jobs. No longer did the manager hear staff complaining about how they went home feeling bad because they couldn't take better care of their patients. Instead they were talking about the nice thank-you cards they received from patients or other ways they had been recognized. Their pride encouraged them to continue making people happy and the unit's culture changed immensely.

The manager had always believed that 'happy employees make happy customers' but now this maxim was reversed to 'happy customers make happy employees.' For years, there had been trouble recruiting but this is no longer the case. The TCU is fully staffed for the first time in five years and overtime costs have decreased as patient satisfaction has increased.

In the fourth quarter, scores rose yet again to 86.9. This marked an eight point increase in one year. The TCU manager was asked to speak to new managers in our multi-hospital system and to the hospital management group about the unit's success. We learned that taking pride in service generates even greater pride in the outcome.

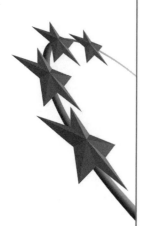

The St. Luke Hospital West

Florence, Ky.

Listening to the "voice of the customer" is important, but as the staff on the pediatric oncology unit at Hackensack University Medical Center learned, it is also wise to listen to the "inner voice" that may suggest it is time to heal those who care for customers. By focusing on the care and comfort of each other, employees on this unit became more effective in responding to the needs of patients and families. In terms of overall satisfaction with nursing care and likelihood to recommend, they moved from being the lowest ranked nursing unit in the hospital to the highest.

Previous to the start of our service initiative, our pediatric oncology nursing unit had a neutral view of the patient satisfaction survey process. Because of the nature of our patient care, we generally assumed that parents just have too much on their minds to worry about completing patient satisfaction surveys. Well, reality hit hard when patient satisfaction results arrived one quarter that rated our 6 Conklin nursing unit the lowest in the hospital for every criterion in the nursing section.

We knew it was time for a change. Not only were our patients' parents responding to the surveys but what they said was not good. So we discarded all of our old, comfortable assumptions. We decided undertake a complete turnaround and pursued feedback from our patients. We knew that their input would be valuable. We wanted to know what they were thinking and feeling so we could begin making a difference.

We reviewed our surveys very carefully, paying special attention to common trends in scoring and to the written comments. Our patients were loud and clear about the areas we should concentrate on. We narrowed our focus to two areas: 1) comfort and convenience for patients and their families, and 2) staff satisfaction and renewal.

Comfort & Convenience for Patients & Their Families. After reviewing surveys, talking with parents and touring each patient room, we brainstormed and implemented several changes. Comfortable lounge chairs were purchased for parents to sleep on. Patient information boards were posted at the bedside to be used to list the patient's daily activities, post messages, and write the name of the nurse with primary responsibility for the child's care each day. Dry-erase boards were placed in each room for the child to write on. Hand-painted murals of comic characters were created in each patient room. A space on the unit was redesigned and turned into a teen lounge. A family lounge was designated for meals, conversation, or just quiet time. With the assistance of the food and nutrition department, a complimentary meal program was established, and a vending machine was placed in the family lounge.

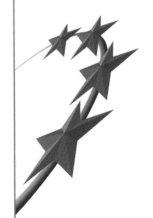

Hackensack University Medical Center

Hackensack, N.J.

45

Staff Satisfaction & Renewal. We realized that we could add all the best conveniences and have the most beautiful environment, but if staff was burned-out or not fulfilled, then all of the other stuff just didn't matter. After all, patient satisfaction is directly related to staff satisfaction.

We began an intense concentration on healing ourselves, as well as our patients. This unfortunately began as a result of a tragedy that happened to a co-worker but the event did bring us together as a team. We began looking at things from different perspectives. The outpouring of kindness and gratitude related to the tragic situation produced respect and collegial compassion toward each other. It has made our job of caring for children with dreaded diseases more bearable. We now take that extra moment to ask team members if they are OK or to offer assistance. We've taken advantage of many support services and improved our own methods of practice to improve staff satisfaction.

Dealing with grief is an unfortunate part of being a staff member of a pediatric oncology unit. Realizing this, the nurse manager has implemented systems of support and guidance that benefit the staff. These programs have provided a safe haven for staff to express their feelings while continuing to provide patient care. The staff of our pastoral care department has held special prayer and reflection sessions for our employees. We've learned better ways to communicate with patients and their family members and more effective ways to express our own frustrations, heartbreaks, and feelings of helplessness.

Every day is a "Pat on the Back" day. We encourage each other by offering compliments and acknowledging each other's efforts and talents. We ask ourselves daily, "Did I give someone a pat on the back today?"

We redesigned our patient care conferences to emphasize nurse/physician communications. We developed a "Friends Award" program that enables us to send certificates to friends and colleagues who have helped us in small or big ways.

All of the hard work paid off. The nursing unit of 6 Conklin went from being rated absolutely last in the hospital for "overall nursing care" and "likelihood to recommend" to first. The overall rating of nursing care increased from 83.5 to 94.3 just one year later. The rating of "likelihood to recommend" increased from 79.4 to 97.2 in a year.

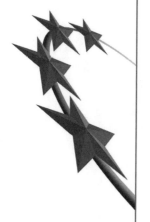

Hackensack
University
Medical Center

Hackensack, N.J.

Research has shown that organizations with engaged employees have higher levels of customer satisfaction. One of the many ways to strengthen employee engagement is to solicit and respond to employee opinions and suggestions. This involvement leads to stronger sense that "I make a difference." When Fairview–University Medical Center, unit 11A, involved employees in soliciting and responding to patients' feedback, it was addressing two important objectives. This approach contributed to the medical center's strategic goals of achieving service excellence and employee engagement throughout the organization.

Unit 11A is the 29-bed medical/surgical/telemetry unit of Fairview–University Medical Center, a 1,868-bed academic teaching hospital in Minneapolis. The unit has approximately 60 employees, including registered nurses, nursing aides, and health unit coordinators. Both academic and community physicians admit patients to the unit. Patients on the unit have a variety of diagnoses, including multiple sclerosis, pneumonia, and gastrointestinal illnesses. Some patients also have mental health and chemical dependency diagnoses.

Staff on patient care unit 11A selected two objectives for the year: 1) create a unit council, and 2) improve customer satisfaction. We wanted to create the unit council because Fairview Health Services, the parent organization of our hospital, had previously released research data that showed a correlation between employee engagement and customer satisfaction.

The institution of our unit council led to a grassroots effort to improve customer satisfaction. This multidisciplinary group reviewed patient satisfaction survey results. They concluded that the "likelihood to recommend the hospital" would be a key indicator of success. Four questions on the satisfaction survey have a high correlation on the likelihood to recommend. These are: 1) staff worked together to care for you (85% correlation), 2) nurses kept you informed (78% correlation), 3) staff sensitivity to inconvenience (70% correlation), and 4) promptness of response to call (69% correlation).

That information, and council members' professional and personal experiences, led to the creation of an elegantly simple plan. We began by asking patients or their loved ones to express what they needed. The admitting nurse is responsible for initiating this dialogue and is aided with by a script. A sign posted each patient room says: *"In order to meet your unique needs, we want to personalize your care while you are here. Please share with us 2 or 3 important things that will help us give you the best possible care. We will write those here for all staff to see when working with you. Please feel free to make changes during your stay."*

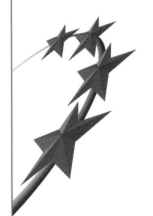

Fairview–
University
Medical Center

Minneapolis, Minn.

47

Patients identified things such as warm blankets, snacks, pain management, privacy, newspapers, pet visits, and timely answering of call lights. Each patient's wishes are written on a board in the room, and staff is responsible for fulfilling those requests to the extent they are able.

Each patient discharged from Fairview–University Medical Center is sent a survey. Unit 11A's mean score on the survey question "Likelihood of your recommending this hospital to others," ranged from 65.9% to 79.0% the year before the customer service initiative began. After the initiative began in March, scores showed a significant increase to 85.2%.

To provide another measure of success, the unit council conducts an informal audit every week. Five patients are randomly selected and asked questions relating to their care. Eighty percent of respondents say caregivers responded to the requests they wrote on the boards. One hundred percent of patients who had been hospitalized elsewhere identify that they had not experienced similar effort by caregivers and 100% respond that our effort made a positive difference in their care.

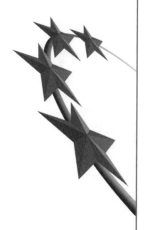

Fairview–
University
Medical Center

Minneapolis, Minn.

Patients' perceptions of the service provided by a department or unit can be changed without spending a lot of money. When the medical-surgical unit at Delaware Valley Hospital found its patient satisfaction scores were only in the 41st percentile nationally, a team was formed, areas with low scores on satisfaction surveys were reviewed, and reasons were investigated. After implementing various low cost solutions, while also communicating more effectively with patients and family members, the unit's overall scores jumped to the 98th percentile.

Delaware Valley Hospital embraced the "Campaign for Excellence" initiative launched by United Health Services, the system to which we belong. We began by creating employee teams to work on achieving goals in specific areas. The Inpatient Satisfaction Team achieved remarkable success by developing and implementing several initiatives that dramatically increased the level of patient satisfaction on our medical-surgical unit within a relatively short period of time.

On learning of our low satisfaction scores, which placed us in the 41st percentile, we were not only shocked but determined to work to improve patient satisfaction as quickly as possible. One of the first initiatives we undertook was to make discharge phone calls. The charge nurse makes calls within 48 hours of discharge to be sure patients understand their discharge instructions and to answer any questions they may have.

The unit manager began making daily rounds to see how patients feel their care has been and to ask if they have any concerns. Staff received communications training and reminders to explain to patients why they were doing things and to demonstrate respect for patient privacy. Note pads were put in the rooms so patients could write questions they wanted answered. Nurses frequently review these notes and either answer the questions or advise physicians so they can respond.

Welcome cards were developed, and these are placed on each bed when rooms are prepared for new admissions. The card thanks the patient for choosing Delaware Valley Hospital for their health care. Housekeepers also leave preprinted cards to inform patients that the room was cleaned while they were away.

Most phone calls incur long distance charges in our rural area, so we now provide phone cards for patients to use. Birthdays and special anniversaries are celebrated by giving patients a card and cake or small gift. Coloring books are available for pediatric patients or young children visiting a family member. A jigsaw puzzle has been set up in the solarium for patients or visitors to piece together.

In deference to the families of deceased patients, we now convey a loved one's personal belongings in a nice tote bag, along with a sympathy card. This

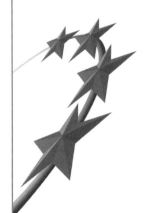

Delaware Valley Hospital
Walton, N.Y.

eliminated the use of plastic bags that gave the impression that we were just throwing a patient's stuff together and getting it out of our way.

Very little has been spent monetarily on this project. The cost of printing cards, providing phone cards and purchasing tote bags has been minimal. Some items for birthdays and anniversaries have been donated by employees, as have the puzzles for the solarium. Many of our initiatives simply involved better communication with both patients and family members.

Great strides have been made in improving satisfaction. The team now has new members and continues to meet regularly. Staff continues to remain aware of what it means to be a patient and how it feels to be "on the other side of the bed." We make a concerted effort to remember to keep patients informed. Improved satisfaction scores and our ranking in the 98th percentile have helped the staff to feel more appreciated and accomplished.

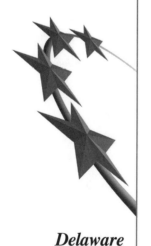

Delaware Valley Hospital

Walton, N.Y.

Customers frequently ignore satisfaction surveys. That is, of course, unless they want to report exceptional satisfaction or dissatisfaction. One of the first things the ambulatory surgery/GI lab at Highsmith–Rainey Memorial Hospital did after naming a Patient Satisfaction Team was to increase the frequency and volume of patient feedback. Employees ask patients to return the satisfaction survey no less than three times before they leave the hospital. The unit also encourages patients to express unmet needs and expectations while they are there, not after they leave. These are just two ways the unit has been able to maintain exceptional customer satisfaction.

The ambulatory surgery/GI lab at Highsmith–Rainey Memorial Hospital receives 10,000 patient visits each year. Patient satisfaction has always been a priority, but once we began receiving patient satisfaction data regularly, our focus became even greater. With the goal to increase and maintain the standards of care and patient satisfaction awareness with a team approach, we assembled a Patient Satisfaction Team.

The team's first task was to increase the return rate of surveys. Our plan of action was to remind patients that their feedback is important to us, and we ask them to return the survey at least three times. The first reminder is given by the nurse when providing discharge instructions. The second reminder is offered by the nursing assistant who escorts the patient out of the hospital. During the post-discharge follow-up call, a third reminder is given. These repetitive requests have succeeded in improving the response rate.

The team decided to make patients feel as if they are entering a friend's home as they enter the unit. Upon arrival to the unit, patients and visitors are greeted with a smile and introduction. The physical environment is inviting and soothing. Staff members wear buttons that say *"We Care"* or *"Just ask me, I will help you!"* Pictures of the staff are posted on the unit's bulletin board, above the caption *"We Care Team."* A comfortable lounge area is available with activities for diversion.

We realize the patient's time is valuable and insist that delays are explained to patients and families in a timely manner. Procedures are explained and patients are encouraged to ask questions. Scripting has enhanced our communications. A few key phrases consistently used are "Is there anything else I can do for you?" and "Did I miss anything?" Introductions follow the protocol of identifying name and title, such as "Hello, my name is Sara and I am your nurse."

Because all staff dress similarly, patients expressed confusion about being able to identify nurses. In response, we placed an extension on all RN badges that reads NURSE. It was a simple fix. The charge nurse conducts rounds with patients and families. During the visits, she specifically asks if the service

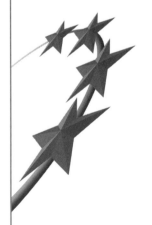

Highsmith–Rainey Memorial Hospital

Fayetteville, N.C.

has been "very good" and whether there is anything more the patients need. We've found that many small but significant issues are addressed as a result of this routine inquiry.

Making patients feel special goes beyond atmosphere and communication, and our ambulatory surgery/GI lab goes the extra mile to provide special services. An express meal is available for patients after their procedures. Coffee is offered to family members while they wait. Parents are encouraged to remain with their children, and family members are permitted to be with their loved ones as much as possible. Pediatric patients are transported in wagons, and age-appropriate videos are available to entertain them. Children are given a stuffed animal to accompany them to the operating room and then home.

We remain sensitive and aware of how we can assure the patient's dignity remains intact. Patients are allowed to keep their dentures unless absolutely contraindicated. Patients are allowed to wear undergarments during procedures that do not involve the lower body. We knock before entering rooms, and we address all patient issues without judgment or condescension.

Framed documents with the name and phone number of the patient care manager are placed in patient rooms. The document reads, *"Our goal is to give 'very good' service. If we have not met this goal, please contact ____ ____ at _____. We would like to hear from you because you make a difference."* If a service breakdown is reported, all staff are empowered to implement the service recovery. The acronym for the program is STAR: Solicit customer feedback, Timely acknowledgement, Apology, Resolution. Soliciting feedback from the patients is usually the only step required.

We continue to care when patients leave our facility. Home care instructions now are placed in a bright orange envelope with the words "DISCHARGE INSTRUCTIONS" printed on the front. We verbally state, "I am placing your home care instructions in the bright orange envelope." Since this action was taken, scores on the survey question relating to "receipt of home care instructions" have increased 2.6 points. The team designed cards thanking the patient for choosing Highsmith–Rainey as their health care provider. These are mailed to patients.

By focusing on learning patient preferences, anticipating and responding to their needs, and encouraging them to return satisfaction surveys, we have achieved high satisfaction scores. The unit is ranked in the 99th percentile in patient satisfaction. Our caring approach to customer service, extended before, during, and after patient encounters, works.

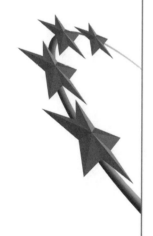

Highsmith–Rainey Memorial Hospital

Fayetteville, N.C.

When the Cancer Center of Cape Fear Valley Health System received its first report from a patient satisfaction survey that had recently been carried out to compare peer institutions, it found that it was ranked in the 36th percentile. The team was in disbelief but after a brief period of denial, they changed their attitudes and accepted the news, but not the results. The staff implemented changes that included extending treatment times and providing recreational activities for patients and family members. The Cancer Center now routinely scores above the 90th percentile nationally in customer service.

The Cancer Center of Cape Fear Valley Health System is comprised of the radiation and medical oncology departments and primarily provides outpatient cancer treatments to approximately 130 to 150 patients a day. Our goal has always been to provide quality, compassionate, and comprehensive care to every patient. Therefore, after the initial shock of learning that we scored in the 36th percentile in patient satisfaction wore off, we moved forward with the goal of exceeding the 90th percentile.

Our journey began when the Cancer Center's employees and physicians attended the "Leading Heroic Service" workshop presented by our health system. Our medical director of radiation oncology's attendance at this session, and his continued support afterward, were demonstrations of his personal commitment to patient satisfaction and to improving the Cancer Center as a whole. This sent a strong message to our staff. After the workshop, a Cancer Center patient satisfaction task force was formed, and it continues to meet regularly. The goal of this group is to brainstorm ideas and to recommend changes related to priority index questions on our patient satisfaction survey. Many changes have occurred as the result of survey feedback from our patients.

Radiation oncology extended treatment times by five minutes per patient in response to the dimension, "wait time in radiation oncology." Previously, patients were scheduled every ten minutes causing patients and therapists to feel rushed. Both therapists and patients gratefully received this change.

Radiation oncology installed privacy curtains in the treatment rooms, simulators, and exam rooms in response to patient feedback on the dimension, "concern for privacy."

Medical oncology created a "Busy Buggy" for patients and families to enjoy while receiving their chemotherapy. The cart is loaded with diversionary activities such as hand-held games, CD headsets, a large variety of music, books on tape, magazines, coloring books, etc. This activity cart was a direct result of the lower scores for the survey question, "things to do while waiting."

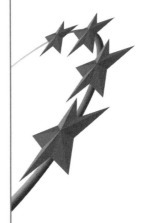

Cape Fear Valley Health System

Fayetteville, N.C.

A social worker now meets with every new patient and family at the beginning of the treatment course to review information about support groups, emotional needs dealing with their relationships, and available resources. Previously, our social worker was meeting with patients on a referral or as-needed basis. This change has resulted in patients feeling more confident and informed by having a specified contact to rely on if assistance is required.

Scripting and "key words" have been incorporated into everything we do. Communicating a consistent message, being aware of body language, and choosing the right words continue to have a positive impact.

A program has been implemented to provide spiritual support to patients who request it. The program was started as an extension of our "Friends of the Cancer Center" volunteer program and has been well received and appreciated by the patients and families who have benefited from the service. Our goal is to be operational Monday through Friday from 8 a.m. to 5 p.m. in order to provide this service when it is needed.

A project we are especially proud of is the Cancer Center Patient Education Handbook. This handbook incorporates information about side effects and symptom management, treatment schedules, staff contacts, support groups, resources, physician and staff qualifications, home care, and more. The handbook encourages patients to participate in their care. This handbook has been a great addition to the many resources we provide to patients, and referring physicians have found it to be a helpful tool.

Education and celebrations have had a huge impact. The entire staff at the Cancer Center has been educated on how to read patient satisfaction reports and understand what the numbers really mean. Satisfaction scores are shared weekly, and patient comments are printed and distributed so that staff can read them. If certain employees are singled out for their dedication or excellence on a survey, they are recognized and thanked. Group celebrations have enhanced teamwork with our ancillary departments.

Everyone who provides services to the Cancer Center is included when we celebrate our success. For the past six quarters, our mean score has not dropped below 90.8, and our percentile ranking has remained above the 90th percentile.

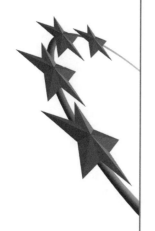

Cape Fear Valley Health System

Fayetteville, N.C.

University of California, Irvine (UCI) Medical Center decided to use a performance improvement approach to improve patient satisfaction scores in its ambulatory care division. Teams targeted for improvement such personal issues as courtesy, promptness, concern, and sensitivity to patient needs. By developing cross-functional teams and strategies to drive the process, they took patient satisfaction from the lowest in the institution to the highest. Since the inception of the customer satisfaction program, ambulatory visits have increased nearly 20%. Despite increased demand, excellence in customer service is making a difference at UCI Medical Center.

UCI Medical Center began focusing on customer service when a new administrative team began to refocus the institution's goals, beginning with a new mission statement that emphasized the importance of quality care, customer satisfaction, and financial value. The chief patient care services officer, the director of pathology services, and the chief ambulatory care officer were charged with developing a patient satisfaction program. A steering committee was formed, along with sub-committees, to gather, analyze, and share data regarding customer perceptions to improve satisfaction within our system and specifically, within the ambulatory care division.

Ambulatory care developed goals around customer service and began making progress and improvement. The steering committee focused on interpersonal issues because those survey questions were consistently listed in the top 10 on the priority list. By focusing on personal issues, we avoided excuses that the aging physical plant was preventing us from attaining our improvement goals. Six survey questions representing those issues included:

- Courtesy of person who scheduled your appointment

- Promptness in returning your phone calls

- Concern the nurse/assistant showed for your problem

- Courtesy of staff in the registration area

- Sensitivity to your needs

- Concern for your privacy

Led by a facilitator from human resources, ambulatory care managers used the medical center's performance improvement model to attack the problems, setting up four performance improvement teams chaired by a nurse manager and consisting of managers, supervisors, staff nurses, medical assistants, and admitting staff from different clinics. Representatives from the call center were included. Each team was given a month to develop strategies to improve customer satisfaction in ambulatory care for the personal issue

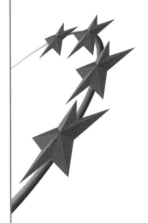

UC Irvine Medical Center

Orange, Calif.

assigned to it. Managers communicated monthly on progress of team efforts. The chief ambulatory care officer met with each clinic at its staff meeting to emphasize the importance this initiative. Scores for ambulatory care and inpatient personal issues are shared monthly at the managers' forum and at staff meetings. Graphic control charts are available on the medical center Intranet for all employees to see. Patient satisfaction quarterly reports are also accessible for managers to review.

When we began this process, our score for likelihood of recommending was 74.6, in the 1st percentile nationally. Five years later, our score was 87.2, in the 57th percentile. With concentration on six personal issues, our score had risen to 77.2 in two years; the score another two years later was 84.5. All ambulatory care physicians, managers, and staff were involved on cross-functional teams. Ambulatory care visits have increased 20%. Given the highly competitive climate in Southern California with managed care dominating the ambulatory service climate, these results are astounding.

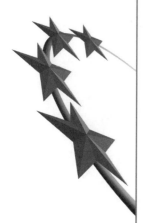

***UC Irvine
Medical Center***

Orange, Calif.

The dietary director at The Toledo Hospital, one of seven hospitals in ProMedica Health System, believed that one of the most important factors influencing quality customer service was employee morale. With this in mind, a Dietary Performance Improvement Team was created. The goal of the team was to create a friendly, compassionate work environment where employees felt respected and valued. In addition to energizing employees and improving customer satisfaction, cafeteria sales increased, attendance improved, and employee turnover decreased.

The Toledo Hospital (TTH) is a tertiary-care hospital with more than 400 beds. The dietary department employs 103 full-time employees and serves more than 990,000 cafeteria and patient meals each year. In keeping with ProMedica Health System's vision to build and support a culture of quality care and superior customer service, a Dietary Performance Improvement Team was established. The goals of the team were to create a friendly, compassionate work environment where employees felt respected and valued and to evaluate every aspect of food service in an effort to improve food quality and customer satisfaction.

The Dietary Performance Improvement Team realized that its efforts to increase the morale of the dietary department would need to be creative and consistent. Initially, the team met several times to brainstorm and discuss ways to keep employees motivated and involved. Several of the morale boosters are simple, obvious ways of saying that we are glad they are a part of the dietary team. For example, small tokens of appreciation or reminders, such as a roll of Life Savers with a tag that says *"We appreciate you a 'hole' lot"* or a dollar coin with a tag that reads *"Our pennies add up to dollars"* are handed out to each dietary employee every month. In addition, monthly discretionary gifts are awarded to individuals who go beyond their job requirements to perform in exemplary ways. Managers frequently write notes of appreciation and mail them to employees' homes when situations arise to recognize acts of kindness or offer positive feedback.

We gave various employees $25 so they could "mystery shop" local restaurants. Participants were required to complete surveys about their experiences and asked to report at monthly staff meetings on how they've incorporated ideas into their own service practices. Customer comments and financial information are shared at monthly meetings. Employees are involved in the interviewing process for supervisors. They sit in on the interview and are encouraged to ask questions and offer feedback. Their opinions are given weight when hiring decisions are made. Employees were involved in the selection of new uniforms. They formed a committee, investigated different options, and made the recommendation for the new uniform. These are just a few of the ideas that have been implemented to show employees that they really do make a difference.

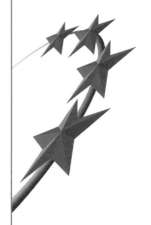

The Toledo Hospital

Toledo, Ohio

Quarterly and annual events are held to reward and/or recognize dietary employees for their service. Fifty dollar gift certificates are given to employees who work a full quarter with perfect attendance. Each year during National Food Service Worker Week, dietary managers serve free meals to dietary employees and raffle off prizes throughout the week. Through various means, every employee is awarded a gift. In the fall, we hold an annual family picnic at a local park, complete with games and clowns. This enables dietary employees and their families to socialize, relax, and enjoy the day.

The second goal of the Dietary Performance Improvement Team was to improve food service and customer satisfaction. The cooks, bakers, salad makers, menu clerks, tray staff, dish washers, and dietitians were asked to evaluate and track every aspect of their jobs. The information was analyzed and trends were noted. Pre-processed frozen and canned entrees were eliminated and replaced with homemade foods that were less expensive, tastier, and lower in sodium. In addition to the cold late tray, a hot alternative is now available. To guarantee consistency of food items, cooks, bakers, and salad makers use the same recipes. Tray delivery times were rearranged to create more flexibility, and floor stock food was individualized on the maternity and children's floors to meet the unique needs of those patients.

The investment required to implement the process improvements and morale boosters was minimal. The return on this investment has been phenomenal. Dietary's turnover rates decreased by almost half the first year, from 30.5% to 19%, and again, to 16.3% the second year. Four years later, staff turnover is 7%. The number of employees with perfect attendance has increased steadily from 1% the first year to an all time high of 23% three years later. Ninety-five percent of respondents to our annual cafeteria survey rated as excellent or good the politeness and friendliness of cafeteria services compared to 88% the year previously. Patient satisfaction scores for overall quality of food posted a statistically significant improvement after dietary process improvements were implemented. The dietary department posted a 10% increase in sales over a twelve-month period.

As astonishing as these figures are, the most impressive indicator of success occurred recently at a monthly department meeting. After presenting the patient satisfaction scores, turnover rates, perfect attendance rates, and cafeteria sales, the dietary employees promptly gave a standing ovation to the director. As the saying goes, "Give credit where credit is due." The dietary director quickly reminded his staff that he only presents the data and they deserved applause for a job well done.

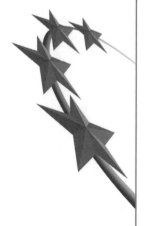

The Toledo Hospital

Toledo, Ohio

During an initiative to provide all patients, family, and staff the best service possible, managers of the department of environmental services at Clara Maass Medical Center, St. Barnabas Health Care System realized a critical link exists between employee and customer satisfaction. A series of steps was taken to ensure that all employees in the department understand that, as housekeepers, they are ambassadors, and they should take pride in their work and recognize their importance to the medical center.

The department of environmental services provides housekeeping services for Clara Maass Medical Center. It is a department that works behind the scenes. The management team has focused on its role in creating a service-driven culture and building employee satisfaction. Our philosophy is that employees are ambassadors and that satisfied employees who feel pride in their work produce valued service for our customers.

We believe this philosophy has contributed to improved employee satisfaction. Based on the most recent employee survey results, our department's scores increased significantly in terms of cleanliness of work environment, respect shown by co-workers, employee attitudes, likelihood that employees would work at the hospital a year from now, and pride felt by our team members. These outcomes are no accident and are a direct result of our initiatives, which have included:

Human Resources. We screen applicants during the interview process in search of those with a customer-orientation.

Conversational Skills. We developed standard scripts for staff to use while interacting with patients and family members. Scripting has provided many of our shy employees with a starting point for engaging dialogue. The standard scripts have been laminated and attached to each housekeeping cart.

First Impressions. We changed the staff uniforms from non-descript attire to a maroon golf shift that clearly identifies the staff as part of the housekeeping department. Each housekeeper now wears his or her new shirt with pride!

Communication. To enhance communications and understanding, we increased the number of staff meetings. We make an effort to foster pride among employees and have found this is beneficial, especially when it comes to preparing for inspections and big projects.

Staff Development. We created a career path for housekeepers who have demonstrated ability to accept additional responsibilities. We have promoted hardworking employees from the ranks into leadership roles by adding several lead positions, and this has been extremely well-received.

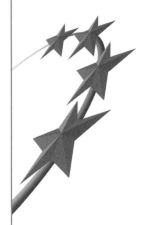

Clara Maass
Medical Center

Belleville, N.J.

Professional Recognition. Although we regularly shower our employees with attention, we take special care to do so during Environmental Services Week by providing meals to employees on all shifts and awarding many prizes and gifts.

Individual Accountability. We post patient satisfaction scores in each janitor closet by the units. After all, they are responsible for their contributions to our department's performance.

Celebration. We celebrate success and use rewards such car wash, dry cleaning, and gift shop certificates and movie tickets to recognize team members.

Involvement. We involve staff and benefit from their expertise when we select equipment and products. We encourage housekeeping managers to participate in professional organizations such as the International Housekeepers Association, and we involve staff on patient satisfaction teams.

Our motto is: *"Take Pride, Take Ownership, Deliver Excellence."*

Our philosophy and approach have won over the employees and performance has steadily improved over time. The improved performance of the department is evident in the steady increase in patient satisfaction for overall cleanliness of the hospital (from 82.2 to 85.5) and courtesy (from 83.9 to 85).

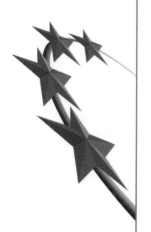

**Clara Maass
Medical Center**

Belleville, N.J.

Studies show that pet companionship has a positive effect on human health and rehabilitation in health care settings. PAWS for Health at Carondelet St. Joseph's Hospital is a program that pairs certified animals with rehabilitation therapists to facilitate patient therapy. The program was initiated to enhance the patient experience and the outcomes of physical and occupational therapies. Since the program began, the average census on the rehabilitation unit and outpatient rehabilitation center has doubled, and patient satisfaction scores are maintained at 96%.

PAWS for Health was initiated at Carondelet St. Joseph's Hospital as the first animal-assisted therapy program in Tucson, Ariz. Local health care organizations in our region have had animal visitation programs, but none had established an animal-assisted therapy program. Studies have shown that pet companionship has a positive effect on human health so this addition to rehabilitation services was a logical step.

The planning and collaboration to design the program began under the leadership of an experienced occupational therapist with extensive experience in dog obedience training and competition. Under her leadership, collaboration began with the Humane Society of Southern Arizona, as well as departments within the hospital.

Policies and procedures were patterned after those established by the Delta Society. Announcement flyers and information about the program were distributed through the local humane society to recruit volunteer pets. The final 15 selected PAWS pets were registered as Pet Partners once they completed a 4-week training program and had at least one year of experience in animal visitation programs to local hospitals, schools, and/or nursing homes. Each handler was oriented through the established hospital volunteer process. Handlers and dogs received photo identification badges. Handlers were given special T-shirts to wear, and we provided bandanas for the dogs. An extensive orientation was held for dogs and handlers to orient them to the rehabilitation process and to discuss and demonstrate the therapy process.

Dogs were scheduled to participate in physical and occupational therapy sessions twice a week. Patients receiving inpatient comprehensive rehabilitation services have the option of including certified therapy animals in their therapy sessions. Patients are interviewed about their experience with animals, any fears, allergies and especially their interest in working with dogs during therapy sessions. Each session is documented to track patient progress, and the variety of therapy activities expands as animal handlers work with therapists to discover how their companion's special skills can be incorporated into each session. A satisfaction evaluation survey is completed by each patient at the end of their PAWS participation.

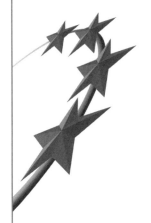

St. Joseph's
Hospital

Tucson, Ariz.

Investment was minimal because of volunteer support. The primary investment has been the salary of the PAWS coordinator and minimal supplies and expenses. All handlers volunteer their time and no additional therapy or support staff was necessary for the program. The return on investment has been incalculable in terms of patient and staff satisfaction, enhanced services, and marketing/public relations opportunities. This program has been the focus of local news station coverage, local newspaper and magazine articles, Humane Society magazine articles, information flyers in veterinarian offices and local obedience classes, and has been included in hospital events such as health fairs, celebrations, and educational presentations. The PAWS pets are welcome at hospital events, and they are always a popular addition.

The key to sustained success is the enthusiastic support of PAWS volunteers. They have a passion for the role of animals in promoting health and well-being and are champions for helping animal-assisted therapy become an accepted practice in Tucson hospitals. We value their opinions and appreciate the time they invest; we invite them to special events and feed special treats to their dogs regularly.

Surveys are administered to all patients at the end of their PAWS participation. Results from patient surveys show 96% to 100% satisfaction. Patient feedback has been tremendous and glowing compliments attest to their appreciation for the service. Employees and animal handler volunteers are surveyed at six-month intervals. Employees extend their full support and volunteers report that they are completely satisfied with the appreciation shown to them and the adequacy of the orientation and education. Average census on the rehabilitation unit and outpatient rehabilitation center has doubled. This program has improved patient and staff satisfaction, and it has made rehabilitation more enjoyable for many people.

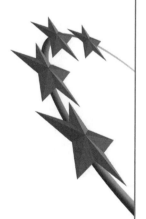

St. Joseph's Hospital

Tucson, Ariz.

CHAPTER 3
SERVICES & SUPPORT

SERVICES & SUPPORT

Transportation remains a significant barrier to health care for the poor. McLeod Regional Medical Center provides services to indigent patients in rural South Carolina. When the McLeod Cancer Clinic realized that transportation issues were resulting in an average of 30 missed appointments a month, the Loving Initiative for Transportation (LIFT) program was launched.

Our small cancer clinic is an outpatient facility serving approximately 200 cancer patients a year, most of whom make regular visits. These patients have no third-party coverage and meet the South Carolina Department of Health and Environmental Control guidelines for financial assistance. We do not charge these patients for the services they receive. They are referred to McLeod's Cancer Clinic by a physician and must have a biopsy-proven diagnosis of cancer.

The clinic is part of McLeod Health, a locally-owned, not-for-profit health system providing services throughout a 12-county region in northeastern and coastal South Carolina. Ours is one of the few remaining programs in the state caring for indigent patients.

Five medical oncologists volunteer their services to support regular monthly clinics. The clinic is dedicated to doing everything we can to help our community win the fight against cancer. The Cancer Clinic is engaged with McLeod's Cancer Center in actively participating on the front-line of cancer education, research, screening, diagnosis, and treatment.

Our clinic was faced with a growing problem that affected the care of many of our patients; too many chemotherapy and radiation appointments were being missed. Although we suspected transportation was a problem, we did not realize how crucial the need really was until we began tracking the number of patients who missed their treatments and the reasons why. We discovered that transportation problems were the cause of about 30 missed appointments every month.

Clinic patients, on average, have to drive 40 miles round-trip for treatments and a few come from as far as 80 miles. One patient had completed five cycles of her chemotherapy but could not complete the sixth and final cycle because she didn't have money to pay a driver.

The Cancer Clinic Team established the goal of providing transportation support that would result in fewer missed appointments and better use of the clinic's resources. The Loving Initiative for Transportation Program (LIFT) began with a $5,000 budget from funds we received from the McLeod Foundation. By design, our initial volume was low because our staff is small and our funds are limited. It made sense to create a manageable program that could be expanded as additional funds were acquired.

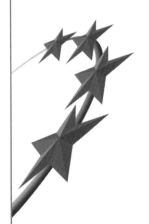

McLeod
Regional
Medical Center

Florence, S.C.

By consulting with local social service agencies, we found a driver who volunteered to provide transportation for 34 cents a mile. The driver is a retiree and he provides similar services for Florence County Department of Social Services. We are working with social service agencies in neighboring counties to identify drivers who can serve as backup.

Many times patients can find someone to bring them to an appointment but they do not have means to compensate the driver. We began distributing $5 and $10 vouchers so patients could purchase gasoline at a local gas station. These vouchers help those who have cars and make it easier for patients to ask for rides from family and friends because they can now reimburse the driver.

Our program is still in its infancy and we continuously seek sources to fund it. To date, we have received $2,500 in additional funds from McLeod Foundation and funds from a national drug company. Recent media coverage resulted in good publicity and the exposure generated many calls from interested parties, including other hospitals inquiring about replicating this program.

McLeod Regional Medical Center's philosophy states that each person is a unique individual, entitled to dignity and respect at all times. While physical needs usually bring the patient to us, their emotional, spiritual, and transportation needs receive our attention as well.

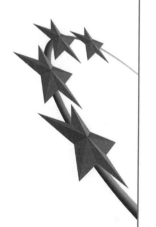

**McLeod
Regional
Medical Center**

Florence, S.C.

Phoebe Putney Memorial Hospital discovered that as many as 15 patients were discharged every month with conditions requiring a ramp at their home. Those without the means to purchase or construct one were forced to make other living arrangements during their convalescence or stay in the hospital. This need gave birth to the Extra Mile Project. Extended stays for homebound patients were eliminated when hospital employees and community volunteers built ramps.

When the director of volunteer services at Phoebe Putney Memorial Hospital (PPMH) heard about a man who had been in the hospital 10 days longer than needed because he could not get into his house, she called the hospital's director of planning. He verified that between three to five patients every month confronted similar barriers and remained hospitalized, at a cost of as much as $1,500 a day per incidence. These two PPMH leaders worked with others within the hospital and community to eliminate the problem.

The Retired Senior Volunteer Program (RSVP) of the Southwest Georgia Council on Aging had started a ramp construction project years earlier to remove a serious safety threat for homebound citizens—the inability to leave their homes because of physical barriers. Dedicated retiree volunteers, ages 62 to 86 years, formed a ramp crew but there was no provision for funding the construction. Some clients paid for their own lumber or made donations, but many were unable to buy even a handful of nails. Through donations of support, 111 ramps were built over a five-year period, but the demand for ramps exceeded RSVP's ability to respond. Ninety percent of the requests for ramps came from PPMH's case managers, physical therapy, home health, and discharge planning staff. RSVP needed manpower and resources. RSVP needed a partner.

The Extra Mile Project, initiated by PPMH employees as a collaborative between PPMH and RSVP, produced an amazing partnership. The project is led by the director of volunteers who first voiced concern for the situation and later crusaded to gain support for the project. Various hospital departments and leaders have been responsible for bringing the project to fruition, including the Community Benefits Committee of the board of directors, administration, and staff from planning, discharge planning, case management, home health, physical rehabilitation, and other departments.

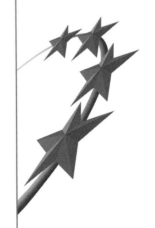

Hospital personnel provided manpower and networking to recruit additional community volunteer crews for ramp construction. For example, the residents from the local Marine Corps base joined together to form the "Ramp America Team." The board's Community Benefits Committee committed $10,000 a year for three years to provide supplies for the construction of "an extra mile" of ramping, which is equivalent to 176 ramps.

Phoebe Putney Memorial Hospital

Albany, Ga.

By increasing volunteers and funding, it has been possible for medically needy homebound citizens to gain freedom from physical barriers and greater access to health care. The first year's results have been stunning as extended lengths of stay for inpatients have been eliminated. The Phoebe Ramp Crew and partnerships with the local Marine Corps base and Lowe's Home Improvement have increased construction manpower by 150%. Although requests for ramps are growing in number, the waiting list has been reduced by 75%.

Contributions to the project increased 200% in nine months. The number of ramps constructed in the first year equaled the total number of ramps built over the previous five years.

Increasing community awareness is an important goal of the Extra Mile Project. The Southwest Georgia United Way gave its highest award, the Volunteer Group of the Year Award, to the Ramp Crew. Ramp crews have been featured in local TV and newspaper coverage. Community awareness for the needs of the homebound is generating new volunteers and donations. People are learning about the service and demand for ramps is growing. The hospital's current strategic plan ensures the project's sustainability. PPMH is committed to identifying and addressing community needs, developing innovative community partnerships, and expanding community health promotion. The Extra Mile Project is this commitment in action.

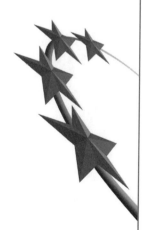

Phoebe Putney Memorial Hospital

Albany, Ga.

Families of patients often have a difficult time locating affordable and convenient accommodations when the hospital is located far from their homes. Carle Foundation Hospital, the hospital auxiliary, and the nearby Amish community formed a unique partnership to ease these separation issues and financial strains by constructing the Carle Auxiliary Guest House. As a free-standing facility that provides warm and inviting accommodations to families of critically ill patients, the Carle Auxiliary Guest House has welcomed more than 2,100 guests since opening.

Carle Foundation Hospital (Carle) serves many critically ill patients of all ages from a 24-county region. The demand for affordable lodging accommodations for families accompanying loved ones to the hospital far exceeded the supply. The Carle Foundation Hospital Auxiliary (Auxiliary) proposed to build or remodel a six-bedroom facility. The Carle board thought the need was much greater and asked the Auxiliary's permission to become a partner in a $1 million project that increased the proposed size to a 12-bedroom house. The Auxiliary expressed the desire to take a major role in the Carle Auxiliary Guest House (Guest House) project, not only by contributing financially but also by donating their time in running day-to-day operations.

A pediatric oncologist who sees Amish patients in his practice suggested that Carle approach the Amish community to build the house. The Amish do not have health insurance and take full responsibility for their health care bills. The cost of major care is often overwhelming. It was suggested that the money saved by contracting with Amish residents could be used to subsidize catastrophic health care costs. When the Amish community agreed, a contract to build the house was signed and construction began.

From the time the Auxiliary first proposed building a guest house there has been excitement within the institution and in the community. The local newspaper and television station regularly echo how dear to the hearts of the community this project is. Local businesses donated or offered reduced prices for building materials. Patients' families have given memorial gifts to purchase furniture, and employees have donated the money they earned while working at Auxiliary fundraisers.

The Auxiliary received support from these communities when it held a successful fundraiser called The Art of Entertaining. The event raised $28,000 and attracted a large number of businesses that expressed interest in sponsoring another event in the future.

The Carle community also became involved. A committee made up of employees from engineering, education, volunteer services, and the clinic, joined members of the Auxiliary and Carle Development Foundation and conducted an employee giving campaign to purchase 12 glider rockers and

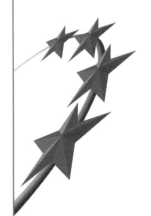

Carle
Foundation
Hospital

Urbana, Ill.

ottomans for the Guest House bedrooms. A rock-a-thon contest between Carle Clinic Association and Carle Foundation Hospital administrators to see which entity could raise more money was one of the highlights of a week-long fundraising campaign. This event, along with sales of donuts, caramel apples and lemon shake-ups, generated funds and created camaraderie among all levels of staff. The goal of $11,000 was exceeded, providing not only the rockers and ottomans but also funds for constructing and furnishing the TV room.

The Operations Committee defined policies and procedures and created a welcome packet for visitors and a referral brochure. The Decorating Committee was charged with furnishing the house in a manner that would be functional, inviting, and user friendly. Considerable thought and care were involved in decisions ranging from the selection of furnishings, linens, colors, and window treatments, to how the kitchen was to be equipped. A party was held to wash and dry 1,391 items such as sheets, pillowcases, towels, and blankets. In late December, the last bed was made and the pantry was stocked in anticipation of the arrival of our first guests.

The day we opened, seven guests were greeted, registered, oriented to the facility, and shown to their rooms. More than 2,100 guests representing 34 states have stayed at the Guest House in the past 18 months.

Since opening the Guest House, volunteers and staff have expressed gratitude for the opportunity to serve families in times of crisis. Everyone has favorite stories about guests they have encountered. The Guest House project continues to garner support from staff, volunteers, visitors and patients alike. Donations from grateful guests average $500 a week. Auxiliary membership has increased 25% since The Guest House opened.

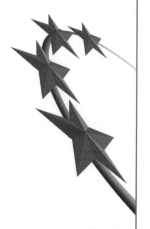

Carle
Foundation
Hospital

Urbana, Ill.

Cultural and language barriers are major challenges for hospitals that provide health care services to diverse patient populations. The Hispanic Patient Educator role was created at Brenner Children's Hospital of Wake Forest University Baptist Medical Center to bridge the linguistic and cultural gaps between Latino/Spanish-speaking patients and the multidisciplinary staff, most of whom are monolingual in English. The Hispanic Patient Educator is a nurse, who has pediatric experience and acts as an interpreter, educator, and advocate.

The Hispanic Patient Educator (HPE) goes beyond the traditional role of an interpreter by incorporating the knowledge and skills of an experienced nurse. The HPE role at Brenner Children's Hospital (BCH) is fulfilled by a registered nurse with pediatric experience who is fluent in Spanish and well-integrated into the Latino culture. The HPE is responsible for inpatient education, staff education, and community outreach.

On patient arrival to the unit, the HPE assists the nursing staff by orienting Spanish-speaking patients and family members to the hospital environment and culture. During the patient's hospitalization, the HPE assists physicians, nurses, and other personnel by explaining medical information to patients and family members. She provides support to the families and makes them feel welcome and cared for. Finally, when these young patients are discharged, the HPE educates parents in post-hospitalization care. The HPE prepares educational materials tailored to meet their needs by performing an assessment of the family's ability to learn and comprehend medical information. Individualized teaching sheets are written that include all of the information necessary for the parents to care for the child at home, such as medication schedules, important phone numbers, follow-up appointments, and care instructions.

The HPE is keenly aware of the barriers encountered by patients and families once they leave the hospital, and she helps parents anticipate problems before they arise. For instance, if a patient is going home to a rural area where medications may not be readily available, the HPE will call the pharmacy before the family leaves the hospital. She helps to narrow communication gaps between outside providers and families of BCH patients who have chronic or serious conditions.

The HPE seeks out opportunities to educate staff about the Latino culture in patient care situations and helps them understand how to overcome challenges when caring for Latino/Spanish-speaking patients.

The HPE developed bilingual admission and intake forms to enable parents to provide necessary information about the personal and medical history of the patient. A proposal is currently under consideration to develop a hospital

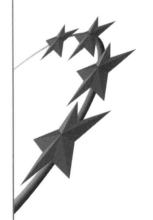

Brenner Children's Hospital

Winston-Salem, N.C.

orientation video in Spanish for the families of children admitted to inpatient units.

Finally, the HPE has a role in the community outside of the hospital. As a bilingual nurse and educator, the HPE participates in health fairs and clinics that reach out to the Latino community. The HPE is an honorary board member of the Ronald McDonald House and a member of the Governor's Task Force for Healthy Carolinians. As a nursing professional, the HPE has been involved with universities locally and abroad to recruit candidates into the nursing workforce at BCH and the North Carolina Baptist Hospital of Wake Forest University Baptist Medical Center. She is currently collaborating with the North Carolina Center for Nursing to attract more young Hispanics into the nursing profession.

Physicians, staff, and patients have reaped the benefits of having a Hispanic Patient Educator. Combining nursing knowledge with Spanish fluency has improved the quality of the hospital stay for Hispanic patients. Patients and family members can verbalize their concerns and questions directly to a member of the health care team without having to use an interpreter. Families find comfort in sharing their concerns with a nurse who understands their cultural and language needs, thus relieving one aspect of the stress that accompanies a child's hospitalization.

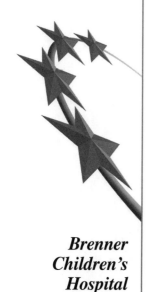

Brenner
Children's
Hospital

Winston-Salem, N.C.

It is often difficult for children who are treated for chronic diseases to keep up with their schoolwork or to assimilate back into the classroom following hospitalization. To combat the impact that illness or disability has on the emotional, social, and educational development of children, La Rabida Children's Hospital developed a tutoring program. Tutoring is provided to patients and their siblings, free of charge.

Giving the gift of learning through our tutoring program enables La Rabida Children's Hospital (La Rabida) to reach out into the community we serve and fulfill our mission as an institution "dedicated to excellence in caring for children with chronic illness, disabilities, or those who have been abused, allowing them to achieve their fullest potential."

The program came to fruition when a young outpatient told his therapist that he needed assistance with his schoolwork. This request led to the conclusion that if one child was looking for help, there must be others among the 5,000 outpatients we serve. A multidisciplinary team with representatives from child life, psychology, social work, and speech pathology was convened to design the program. Each child attends a one-hour session each week and is assigned one tutor with whom to work throughout the school year. More than 25% of the volunteers are La Rabida employees and others are community volunteers. Sessions are offered two days a week in the evenings throughout the academic school year. The budget for the program is less than $9,000, with the majority of funds spent on snacks provided at each of the sessions. The program is funded through La Rabida's in-kind donations and by a private donor.

The tutoring program has grown by leaps and bounds in just three years and is an essential resource in helping our children and their siblings reach their maximum potential, raising their possibilities for a lifetime. We believe that this is the only free, hospital-based tutoring program for outpatient children and their siblings in the country. One hundred percent of the parents and caregivers are satisfied and 90% affirm that it has had a positive effect on their child's performance in school.

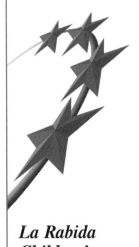

La Rabida Children's Hospital

Chicago, Ill.

Alleviating fear of the unknown can help patients prepare for surgery. This is particularly true in pediatric cases, when both child and parent experience anxieties about the upcoming event. The KIDZ Program at Columbia Memorial Hospital is a perioperative teaching program for children and their parents. The purpose of the program is to reduce fears and stress that are intrinsic to the surgical experience.

The KIDZ Program prepares both children and parents for surgery and incorporates all phases of the surgical experience, from entering the doctor's office to being discharged from the hospital. The surgeon's office staff arranges the appointment for the one hour tour held at Columbia Memorial Hospital.

On arrival, the program coordinator greets the child and parent(s) and begins interacting with the child to assess his or her capacity for understanding. This assessment influences how communications will be conducted. The child is then donned in surgical attire, including a mask, cap, booties and hospital cover-up. The coordinator conducts a "walk through" of the perioperative departments and explains the equipment and procedures. Children and parents are introduced to the operating room and are shown the tables, lights, scrub sinks, and anesthesia equipment. The child is encouraged to ask questions and touch various pieces of equipment.

On the morning of surgery, efforts are made to assign the same surgical staff to care for the child. Typically, 90% of our elective surgical pediatric patients are discharged the same day. Follow-up telephone calls are initiated 1-2 days post-operative. Our patient satisfaction surveys reveal positive responses by the parents and children who attend this preliminary educational session. Since starting the KIDZ Program, we've seen an increase in referrals to the program from surgeons. We also noted a 38% increase in pediatric ambulatory surgery cases in one year. The popularity of the program has resulted in schools requesting participation in tours as a learning activity.

As a community hospital in a small city, we understand patients appreciate knowing who will be caring for them. The pre-surgical experience has enabled parents to feel more comfortable while anticipating and planning for their child's elective surgery.

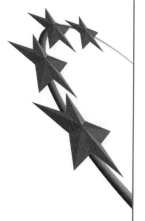

Columbia Memorial Hospital

Hudson, N.Y.

Cancer patients are frequently overwhelmed by the schedule and effects of oncology treatments and frustrated by difficulties finding products they need. The Ellen H. Lazar Shoppe on Fifth was established by Hackensack University Medical Center to provide quality products in a private setting for patients who are undergoing or have completed treatments for cancer.

Professionals who work with cancer patients acknowledge that products and services aimed at improving self-image and quality of life make a difference in how patients cope with their diagnosis and treatment. Hackensack University Medical Center conceived a specialty retail shop designed to enable patients to purchase what they need to improve their lives while undergoing rigorous treatments.

We determined that patients with breast cancer would probably be the store's primary customer group. Data revealed almost 25% of all patients diagnosed with cancer in any given year at HUMC are diagnosed with breast cancer. Patients with breast cancer, in particular, face several cosmetic changes— they may lose one or both breasts and/or the treatment can cause them to lose hair or result in skin problems. A survey of physicians and patients helped planners decide which types of products to carry.

The Shoppe is located down the hall from the Betty Torricelli Institute for Breast Care on the fifth floor of Hackensack University Medical Center's Medical Plaza. The shop offers a warm ambience that is a welcome departure from the typical environment of most hospital-based retail outlets. From state-of-the-art breast prostheses to scarves and handbags, the Shoppe is an oasis for cancer patients who may have a difficult time finding the special products they need.

The Shoppe required an investment of $250,000 and opened in February 1999. It was officially named the Ellen H. Lazar Shoppe on Fifth when an endowment from a memorial foundation provided the opportunity to serve a wider community of women by offering confidential services and free products to the underinsured.

At the Shoppe, women are fitted for a breast prosthesis and they can acquire clothing and other products that will disguise or lessen the effects of their cancer treatments including swimwear, wigs, lymphedema sleeves, skin care products, accessories, and materials such as books, tapes and videos. Although the Shoppe focuses primarily on the female oncology patient, men and children are not excluded. Bedside visits are made by the Shoppe's staff or trained volunteers so patients who are not able to come into the store can learn about the products and services.

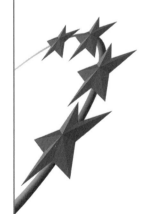

Hackensack University Medical Center

Hackensack, N.J.

A checklist completed during a prosthesis fitting has enabled the staff of the Shoppe to compile a file of consumers that includes their purchases and preferences. The checklist also serves as a means by which the fitter can communicate with the customer to build a strong repeat-customer base. The checklist contains an area for physician referral information, and a letter is sent to the physician with information regarding the Shoppe and its products, as well as Medicare reimbursement and coding criteria. Each patient is given a *"Coping"* magazine and the Shoppe's panel card which offers a discount for future purchases. In addition, each customer is asked to complete a brief customer satisfaction response card.

We are proud that the Shoppe received recognition by earning the highest score of any outpatient department at HUMC for "likelihood to recommend." By listening to our customers, we are able to discover ways to improve and expand our services. We are motivated by the desire to serve and we treat the clients as the valuable assets they are to our specialty store. We are committed to fulfill our roles with integrity and responsibly use our resources to contribute to HUMC's "Bond of Caring."

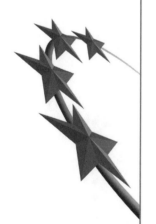

Hackensack University Medical Center

Hackensack, N.J.

The combination of traditional western medicine with therapeutic arts is a fast-growing trend that contributes to the comprehensive care of patients. Innovations in Healing–Using the Arts explores the value of therapeutic arts to promote a culture of healing in a public hospital setting, and honors the ethnicities and traditions of the diverse, multi-cultural populations receiving and providing care at Harbor–UCLA Medical Center.

The Center for Clinical Practice, Education and Research in the Medical Arts at Harbor–UCLA Medical Center was established by organizational and community leaders who were inspired by the growing popularity of therapeutic arts in health care.

The objectives of the center's Innovations in Healing–Using the Arts program are to: 1) create a culture of healing through the arts and the environment, 2) establish a risk-taking environment that uses innovation as a "norm" to bridge cultural, informational and communicative gaps between the patient, family, and health care team, 3) recognize how creative expression through visual and performance arts can promote patient and staff appreciation of cultural commonalities and differences, and 4) explore the use of the arts to promote communication, participation, collaboration, and esprit de corps between Harbor–UCLA and its community. Core activities revolve around three areas of focus:

Artists in Residence. Harbor–UCLA utilizes local artists to work with hospitalized patients. These artists exhibit their work at the hospital and present open seminars to hospital staff and the public regarding their views on their own work and its personal and/or societal relevance.

Music in the Plaza. The center sponsors a series of performances on the campus to give patients and staff opportunities to enjoy a wide range of musical and theatrical recitals.

Campus and Hospital Arts Beautification. The hospital's structure and environment have been beautified with murals, sculptures, paintings, photography, and a labyrinth that is believed to be the first of its kind situated in a hospital setting.

The success of our Innovations in Healing–Using the Arts program is the result of participants on our team who donate their time, effort, and resources to creating a culture where healing, art, and creativity flourish. With the support of Harbor–UCLA's progressive leaders, the team has been empowered to create a campus where art and healing are integrated with science and technology.

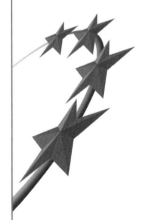

Harbor–UCLA
Medical Center

Torrance, Calif.

The basic theory of music as therapy is that it helps people relax. Seeking to enhance the clinical aspect of medicine with the healing properties of music, St. Bernardine Medical Center initiated a Music Ministry program and discovered that music delivers many more benefits than simply calming patients and easing stress. The outcomes have verified numerous studies supporting music as a component of the healing process.

Hans Christian Andersen said, "Where words fail, music speaks," and at St. Bernardine Medical Center we have incorporated one of the oldest and most holistic of medical approaches into the state-of-the-art care we offer patients. Combined with traditional medicine, clinical expertise, and compassion, our Music Ministry program is a tool we use to lessen the physiologic and psychologic impact of illness and injury on our patients.

Scientific data support the benefits of music in health care. One study found that people who listened to music before surgical procedures experienced reduced blood pressure and pulse rates and less pre-operative anxiety and post-operative pain. Another study observed that those who listen to music during surgery require less anesthesia, experience reduced blood loss, and require less pain medication after surgery.

The opportunity to offer a non-invasive, healing method for our patients was the catalyst behind our Music Ministry program. Initially funded with a $26,000 grant from the St. Bernardine Medical Center Foundation, a bi-lingual vocalist began visiting patients three times a week.

The initial outcomes were remarkable and verified multiple studies supporting music as a component of the healing process. Dying patients felt comforted; patients who had not spoken a word in weeks suddenly made sounds in response to the music; blood pressures stabilized; rapid breathing slowed; less pain medication was requested; and babies in the neonatal intensive care unit ceased crying. An unexpected outcome was the benefit it provided to our employees and especially those working in intensive care and oncology areas of the hospital.

The successes of our initial program allowed us to add two harpists, thereby offering music five days a week. We are producing a musical CD featuring some of the most requested songs to give to patients when the vocalist is not available. Every day with music brings a new story of reduced pain, less stress, or enhanced comfort provided by our musicians. After listening to a harpist's version of Gershwin's *"Someone to Watch Over Me,"* an 80-year old patient exclaimed, "That's what I need, someone to watch over me!"

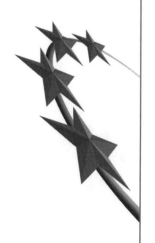

St. Bernardine Medical Center

San Bernardino, Calif.

Life is full of stories and recounting those stories can evoke laughter or tears—and sometimes both. Numerous scientific studies suggest that emotions associated with memories and experiences impact health, and thus, stories can be a powerful healing medium. Mountain States Health Alliance brings renowned and accomplished storytellers into patients' rooms through video broadcast of *Stories for the Soul.*

A number of individuals in our community saw the important link between stories and healing and graciously donated funds to create *Stories for the Soul.* This collection of 11 videotaped stories, as told by professional storytellers and filmed before a live audience at the International Storytelling Center (ISC) in Jonesborough, Tenn., illuminates positive imagery and helps to capture healing moments for the benefit of patients and families.

To our knowledge, *Stories for the Soul* is the only video series of its kind created especially for use in a health care setting. Fourteen storytellers from across the country were each invited to spend a week in Jonesborough as the ISC's resident storyteller. Visitors to ISC were delighted by the opportunity to hear these storytellers perform. Sessions were videotaped, edited, and placed on the in-house television network at Mountain State Health Alliance's (MSHA) flagship tertiary facility, Johnson City Medical Center.

Expansion of the programming is underway within other MSHA facilities. Our drive for the success of this program has become so prominent that funding was again provided by members of the community. This year, 22 resident storytellers are being taped for a sequel series.

Further integration of storytelling in the health care setting is being undertaken through workshops that teach caregivers storytelling techniques. Stories can be used to help relieve stress in the workplace.

In her book, *"Awakening Intuition,"* Mona Lisa Schulz, M.D., underscored the importance of the emotional umbilical cord in health care and the use of approaches similar to those used in *Stories for the Soul.* Leland Kaiser, Ph.D., a well-known health care futurist, recommends the use of healing stories and humor in patient care to increase immunity levels and provide hope and direction to bored or depressed patients. MSHA's collaboration with the ISC contributes to patient-centered care and represents our commitment to excellence.

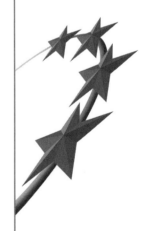

*Mountain States
Health Alliance*

Johnson City, Tenn.

Families of critically ill patients have needs that are often overlooked due to the intensity of their circumstances. Johnson City Medical Center recognized that families in crisis have special needs and in response developed the Family Advocate program. Family Advocates help to facilitate communication, provide reassurance, and care for families while nurses and physicians care for their loved ones.

Caring for families in crisis is the cornerstone of the Family Advocate program. The program was initially designed by Johnson City Medical Center (JCMC) in response to the needs of families of patients in critical care units. The advocate role expanded as the program grew to encompass the emergency room, cardiac cath labs, and main surgery waiting areas.

All families with loved ones in critical care units have access to a Family Advocate 24 hours per day. Advocates are members of the code team and are summoned to respond in those situations. Advocates are paged when trauma patients are brought to the hospital so they can be available when family members arrive at the emergency department. In surgery waiting areas, Advocates relay information to waiting family members and notify them when surgeons are ready for post-surgical conferences.

Advocates organize and coordinate services with the needs of the family in mind. They handle JCMC's innovative "Be Our Guest" program that links those from outside the city to hotels, restaurants, houses of worship, and services in the community.

Patient satisfaction related to interactions with Family Advocates continues to score in the top quartiles. The number of compliments is at an all time high, and the number of complaints related to issues within the Family Advocate scope has fallen precipitously.

We believe caring for family members strengthens the family's capability to support and care for the patient. JCMC's budget to support this program is approximately $300,000. The program proved so successful that it is being implemented in other Mountain States Health Alliance facilities. It is one more way that Mountain States Health Alliance is bringing loving care to health care.

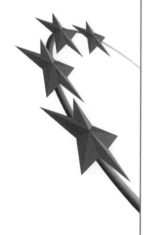

Mountain States Health Alliance

Johnson City, Tenn.

80

A leadership team at Capital Health District Authority in Nova Scotia, organized an interdisciplinary advisory council to validate that high tech and high touch can and do co-exist in a critical care practice environment. The council is advised by former patients and family members. The council members continuously seek ways to care for and support family members, as well as patients. This council has been responsible for the development of several patient/family care initiatives.

As clinicians and providers of critical care to patients, we were interested to view patient care through the eyes and experiences of patients and families. With the help of patients and families advising our Critical Care Patient – Family Council, we developed programs to improve our sensitivity and responsiveness to their needs.

We established a communication link with families by using pagers to keep them apprised of their loved ones' conditions, allowing them greater independence and mobility. Survey results indicate that 87% of the ICU families found these pagers decreased their anxieties and 82.8% reported the enhanced communication caused them to feel more participative as a member of the patient care team. We recruited volunteers to act as non-medical liaisons and offer support and comfort to ICU families. We created a "Family Care Kit" to ensure that families have personal items they need to be more comfortable. We developed a new model to improve end-of-life care, and we offer special support to families of organ donors.

We also asked family members to share stories of their experiences and perceptions when loved ones were transferred from our care to acute care units. We used these insights while mapping how to make that transition seamless and more positive. A chaplain and a social worker are now assigned to the ICU to help families cope with crisis and create more supportive and positive experiences.

In contrast to the sterile world of the ICU, the waiting room now incorporates attributes of warmth, sensitivity, and spirituality thanks to the suggestions of our advisors and council members.

We encourage families to write about their ICU experiences. The entries in these reflective journals are testimonials to the strength, resilience, hope, and faith that are necessary to endure the difficulties of threatening illnesses.

The Critical Care Patient – Family Council has helped us to adopt a paradigm shift in adult critical care, and we are privileged to view our service through the lens of their experiences.

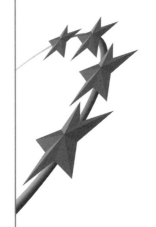

Capital Health
District Authority

Halifax, Nova Scotia

A growing body of literature explores the relationship between patients' spiritual needs and the clinical aspects of their medical care. At Clara Maass Medical Center, Clinical Pastoral Education is used to train clergy to address the spiritual needs of patients, family members, and hospital staff. Initial results show that increased use of trained clergy is positively contributing to patient satisfaction.

C linical Pastoral Education (CPE) is used to train clergy for chaplaincy in health care. On arrival at Clara Maass Medical Center (CMMC), the director of pastoral care reinitiated an intensive CPE training course and recruited five new chaplain interns to participate.

There is a growing demand for professionals who are trained in CPE. The CPE program brings theological students and ministers of all faiths (pastors, priests, rabbis, imams, seminarians, and others) into encounters with persons who are ill or in crisis. The intense involvement with persons in need, as well as feedback from peers and supervisors, help CPE students develop a new awareness of themselves as individuals and the needs of those to whom they minister.

As part of the CPE course work, chaplains were assigned to specific units of the hospital. Group therapy exercises, group interactions, evaluations and sharing were methods used in CPE education. Students were encouraged to recognize their differing gifts for ministry and how those gifts could be shaped and improved. Patient, family, peer, staff, and supervisor encounters introduced challenges which lead to growth and development.

The excellent training that has been provided to chaplains at CMMC and the increased level of responsiveness to patients' needs encouraged by staff referrals to chaplains have contributed to improved patient satisfaction. Performance rankings improved 35% to 90% on various units once CPE-trained chaplains were put into place throughout the medical center. The department of pastoral care received a certificate of recognition, acknowledging the department's attainment of the most improved patient satisfaction score of all departments at CMMC.

In 1950, Helen Flanders Dunbar, M.Div., Ph.D., chair of the Department of Psychiatry at Columbia Presbyterian Medical Center, identified through research that patients who had meaningful interventions with clinically trained chaplains, as compared with those who did not, left the hospital sooner, healed more rapidly, and lived longer. This research conducted over 50 years ago supports our decision to provide trained clergy to respond to patient and family needs at CMMC.

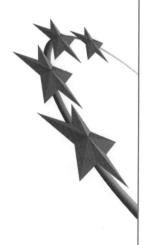

Clara Maass Medical Center

Belleville, N.J.

Providing comfort to families who have lost loved ones is an extension of the caring support provided by hospice staff. By turning a garment worn by a deceased loved one into a cuddly bear, dedicated volunteers at Sharp HospiceCare help to preserve memories and offer comfort to those who are grieving. Since the inception of the Memory Bear program, more than 400 bears have been delivered to appreciative families.

The Memory Bear Program at Sharp HospiceCare was designed as a way for hospice staff to reach out to bereaved families. The cuddly bears are made from a piece of clothing or another sentimental fabric swatch left behind when a loved one passes away.

Initially, eight volunteers were trained to make the bears, but due to the popularity of the program, more were needed. Sharp contacted community groups throughout San Diego to participate and recruited women from three quilting guilds, a cloth doll society, and the American Association of University Women. Today, more than 30 volunteers are now using garments provided by families and loved ones to create these unique keepsakes.

The program has had greater impact than anyone ever envisioned. The NASA Astronauts Spouse Group in Houston, Texas, heard about the program and has been in touch with the program coordinator to have bears made for the surviving family members of the 2003 Columbia crew, as well as the 1986 Challenger crew. Garments sent by the family of a Challenger astronaut have been made into four bears and returned to the astronaut's widow and her grown children.

The bears are gifts to loved ones and it is touching to witness their reactions when they hold the bears for the first time. One person wrote this poem after receiving her bear:

> *Clothing that you once would wear,*
> *Has now become my memory bear.*
> *So when I feel sad or just want to cry,*
> *I pick you up; I know you're close by.*
> *I hold you close and just think of you,*
> *Smiling at me and hugging me too!*
> *I set you back down and then crack a smile.*
> *I feel happy again, if just for awhile.*

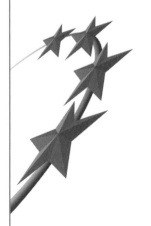

Sharp HospiceCare

San Diego, Calif.

Bereavement programs provide needed support to those who survive a loved one. St. Francis Hospice conceived a way to help grieving survivors get back on their feet, by creating Walk in the Mall. The goal is to provide a safe environment where survivors can gather, share their grief and achieve well-being and stress reduction through physical exercise. The activity, held at local shopping malls, is so popular that 90% of more than 1,500 survivors have participated for over two years.

Established in 1978, the St. Francis Hospice—an entity of the St. Francis Health Care System of Hawaii—is the oldest and the largest hospice in the state of Hawaii. The hospice provides a specialized health care milieu where terminally ill patients, from infancy to more than 100 years of age, spend their last days. Patients are able to remain at home, or they stay in our hospice inpatient facilities, The Sister Maureen Keleher Center in Honolulu or the Maurice J. Sullivan Family Hospice Center in Ewa Beach, where they die free of pain.

An integral part of our program is the bereavement services we provide to family survivors. We make follow-up calls and visits to assess their grief needs after the death and send supportive letters monthly and at appropriate times during the year, such as anniversaries and holidays. In addition, we invite the survivors to regular grief workshops, support groups, and social functions such as picnics and potluck gatherings. When requested, we provide grief education to agencies, schools, churches, nursing homes, and other organizations throughout the island of Oahu. The demand for bereavement services from our survivors, as well as from the community, has increased dramatically.

We developed Walk in the Mall to give survivors the chance to meet regularly to receive the benefits of exercise, re-socialization and grief support. We sponsor five walks a month at alternating malls, and more than 1,500 walkers participate. Registered nurses are available to perform blood pressure and pulse checks. Walkers with abnormalities are referred to physicians. More than 90% of the survivors who attend the weekly walks have been participating regularly for the past two years. As a result of our walks and associated bereavement services, many survivors have become bereavement volunteers who now comfort the newly-bereaved. These programs fulfill our mission to provide a community-based continuum of health related services to the people of Hawaii under the Franciscan values of peacemaking, simplicity, charity, and joy.

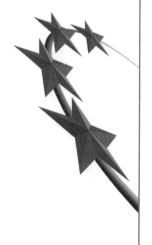

St. Francis Hospice

Honolulu, Hawaii

Because We Care, a family bereavement program at Brenner Children's Hospital, was first envisioned by two pediatric staff nurses in response to the intense needs of parents at the time of and following their child's death. From this vision, a multidisciplinary team approach to bereavement support evolved. Fewer than 1% of the parents who receive materials about the program request no further contact, and more than 100 families a year avail themselves to the services and support.

The goal of the Because We Care (BWC) program is to provide parents and families with emotional support, literature, and awareness of available bereavement resources after the death of a child. The program has become an extension of the skilled and loving care the staff at Brenner Children's Hospital (BCH) provides to all patients and their families.

This program is offered to all parents who have lost an infant or child at BCH. In order to maintain continued support, a member of the health team contacts the family at specific intervals for a minimum of one year. Members of the team include nurses, physicians, child life specialists, social workers, chaplains, and other health care professionals. Follow-up includes telephone contact, handwritten notes, cards, and literature tailored for that individual family.

Between 95 and 120 families receive support each year. Holidays, the child's birthday, and the first anniversary of a child's death are extremely difficult times for grieving parents. These are scheduled contact intervals, and over the course of a year the parents will hear from us 8 to 10 times. BCH typically has between 95 and 120 bereaved families receiving support each year.

Every December, BCH holds a special service to honor the memory of children who have died at our hospital. Family, friends, and staff gather to remember and celebrate the lives of these children. The BWC committee decorates a memorial tree with a star for each child.

Program education is vital, not only for volunteers who maintain contact with bereaved families, but for other staff within BCH and throughout the Wake Forest University Baptist Medical Center (WFUBMC). We have produced orientation and training videos and we maintain a resource library with tapes and books. Educational sessions are routinely scheduled, as is an annual conference. This day-long event focuses on issues specific to "what we do... whether caring for and supporting our special patients and parents or taking care of and nurturing ourselves."

BWC was initially funded by the Friends of Brenner Children's Hospital, a volunteer non-profit community organization. The pediatrics department has now become the major source of financial support. Additional donations of money and services have been provided by many local groups and orga-

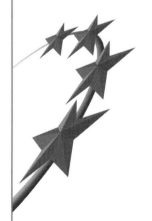

***Brenner
Children's
Hospital***

Winston-Salem, N.C.

nizations such as schools, church youth groups, and adult fellowships, artists and agencies, individuals, and families.

BWC education extends beyond WFUBMC to the broader spectrum of the health care community and the community at large. The program manager provides education to students from several area nursing programs and is an active member and resource for the Pediatric Community Alliance (PCA), organized by our local hospice. PCA is a group of community individuals and organizations committed to facilitating vision and growth among advocates of care for infants and children living with life-threatening conditions and their families. In addition, PCA offers extended bereavement care and support.

Feedback received from evaluations, letters, and telephone calls, reinforces that the program is meaningful and helps to identify ways we can strengthen our support. A release form is provided to families after 4 to 6 weeks, asking if they would like to participate in this program or prefer not to be contacted again regarding support. Providing families with this form and a stamped, self-addressed envelope makes it easy for parents to complete and return. Fewer than 1% of parents request no further contact.

In this day of family-centered care and community outreach, BWC has become an extension of the skilled and loving care the staff at BCH provides to all families. We are given a remarkable opportunity to continue that caring and emotional support after a patient dies. Knowing that others remember their child is a tremendous source of comfort to bereaved parents, and that is what the program is all about. We listen, we care, and we support our families. We remember our patients and our remembering makes a difference.

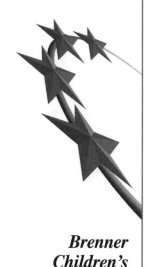

Brenner
Children's
Hospital

Winston-Salem, N.C.

Rituals, combined with bereavement counseling, help to ease the pain of parents who experience perinatal losses while in the care of Harrisburg Hospital. The Perinatal Bereavement Services Program is an insightful model of care that has helped PinnacleHealth System extend support to more than 500 patients who have experienced miscarriage, stillbirth or death of a newborn.

The perinatal bereavement support offered to parents gives Harrisburg Hospital the opportunity to demonstrate PinnacleHealth System's mission to provide compassionate, quality care, and concern for the well-being of others. Women who experience perinatal loss need to heal emotionally, as well as physically. Our program addresses her needs and those experienced by fathers and families.

Led by a clinical nurse specialist, an interdisciplinary team at Harrisburg Hospital developed the creative model of care and services for bereaved parents. We collaborated with agencies and volunteer groups in the community to enhance and personalize our perinatal bereavement services. For example, a local artist makes memory boxes to give to each mother who has lost a baby. The mother can place a lock of the baby's hair, footprints, or a picture in the beautifully decorated memory box to help her remember the child. A women's group knits blankets and baby hats so mothers can swaddle and hold their infants and keep the blanket and hat as keepsakes.

Another example of collaboration is the arrangement we established with a local funeral home to offer cremation for early fetal deaths at no cost to the parents. Cremains are presented in flannel pouches that are made by a local women's group. PinnacleHealth arranges for unclaimed ashes to be interred at a local cemetery.

A local SHARE support group offers ongoing support. A community memorial garden was donated as a place for parents to go to peacefully reflect. An annual "Walk to Remember" is held in October as a memorial to the babies who died during the year.

The program would not be successful without the participation of caring employees who refer families and those who counsel them. Parents receive individualized follow-up, counseling, and support from one of 12 RN bereavement counselors. To be selected and trained as a RN bereavement counselor, each candidate must submit an introspective questionnaire, resume, and application. Candidates are then interviewed and selected by the nurse manager and the clinical nurse specialist. They complete a two-day "Resolve through Sharing" workshop to develop bereavement counseling skills. Additional in-services are conducted for maternity, outpatient surgery, emergency room, and neonatal intensive care staff, and for local chaplains, social workers, and educators.

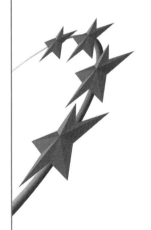

PinnacleHealth

Harrisburg, Pa.

An advisory committee consisting of nurses, a physician, social worker, a member of pastoral care, and a funeral director has been formed to guide and direct the program going forward.

Patients and families comment on the significance of the care they receive. Counselors state that their role is rewarding and fulfilling. Staff nurses report feeling better prepared to care for patients as a result of the training they receive. The knowledge that we have helped a family through a most difficult event and started them on a course of healing is the best reward we can receive.

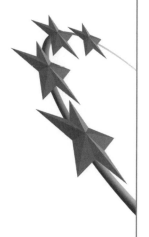

PinnacleHealth

Harrisburg, Pa.

The bonds created between patients, families, and staff are often abruptly severed when patients are discharged from critical care units. Imperial Point Medical Center invites former Intensive Care Unit patients to return to the hospital for an annual party called "Champion Celebration." Patients, families, and the ICU staff are given the opportunity to reunite and to celebrate their shared victories.

For the first annual Champion Celebration sponsored by Imperial Point Medical Center, invitations designed by the intensive care unit (ICU) staff were sent to former patients, inviting them and their families to the celebration. Planned as a special evening to celebrate the human spirit, the event was held in the hospital's cafeteria.

On their arrival, patients received blue ribbons, identifying them as "champions." They also received a swatch of fabric on which to write a message of hope to inspire others who face life-threatening challenges similar to what they confronted. These swatches were then quilted together to make a Critical Care Champion Quilt. The highlight of the event the following year was the unveiling and blessing of this quilt, which now hangs in the ICU waiting room, lending hope and love to all who wait.

"As nurses, we must look at pain and suffering often, but it is wonderful to be given the opportunity to look into the eyes of former patients and see gratitude and love," said Margaret Winters, RN, who chaired the planning of the inaugural event. She then concluded, "It is a wonderful evening; a time when we, as nurses can see the fruits of our labor, and patients are given the opportunity to celebrate the strength of the human spirit. To care for patients in their time of crisis is our challenge as nurses. To celebrate hope, love, and courage with them is our blessing."

The success of the Champion Celebration can be measured by the number of complimentary letters and comments received, though its real success is woven into the swatches of fabric that form the quilts. With plans to sponsor champion celebrations annually, future quilts will decorate ICU patient rooms and offer hope to many for years to come.

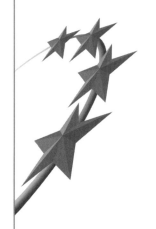

*Imperial Point
Medical Center*

Fort Lauderdale, Fla.

As they confront illness, disability, or the end of life, residents of long term care facilities benefit from programs and activities that address their spiritual needs and cultural orientations. Spiritual programs help residents of Daughters of Israel find solace in their culture and Jewish religion through music, stories, and dance.

Programs and activities enhance the daily lives of our residents. "Spirituality Programs Acknowledging, Revitalizing, and Kindling Souls" are known at the Daughters of Israel as SPARKS. This program incorporates several cultural components:

At My Mother's Knee. Certain religious and cultural impressions are made at a very young age, often at home within the comfort and warmth of the family. These memories include Yiddish expressions, key prayers, Jewish songs, and the smells and tastes of a holiday meal. At My Mother's Knee seeks to elicit these memories through monthly programs that include songs, cooking, discussions, and rituals.

Baby Brigade. Nothing brings a smile to a resident's face faster than a baby. Parents in the community bring their young children to interact with residents in an intergenerational program that brings joy to all who are involved.

Bikur Cholim Volunteers and One-to-One Counseling. In conjunction with MetroWest Jewish Health and Healing Center, volunteers are paired with residents who are considered to be at risk for depression or isolation. Additional counseling is provided by our Interdisciplinary Care Team.

We train our staff to properly assist residents with holiday celebrations. Through formal training sessions, contests, and handouts, our employees are educated about Jewish culture and heritage so they will understand the significance of each holiday in the eyes of Jewish residents.

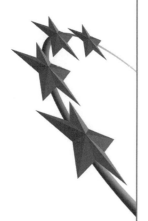

**Daughters
of Israel**

Orange, N.J.

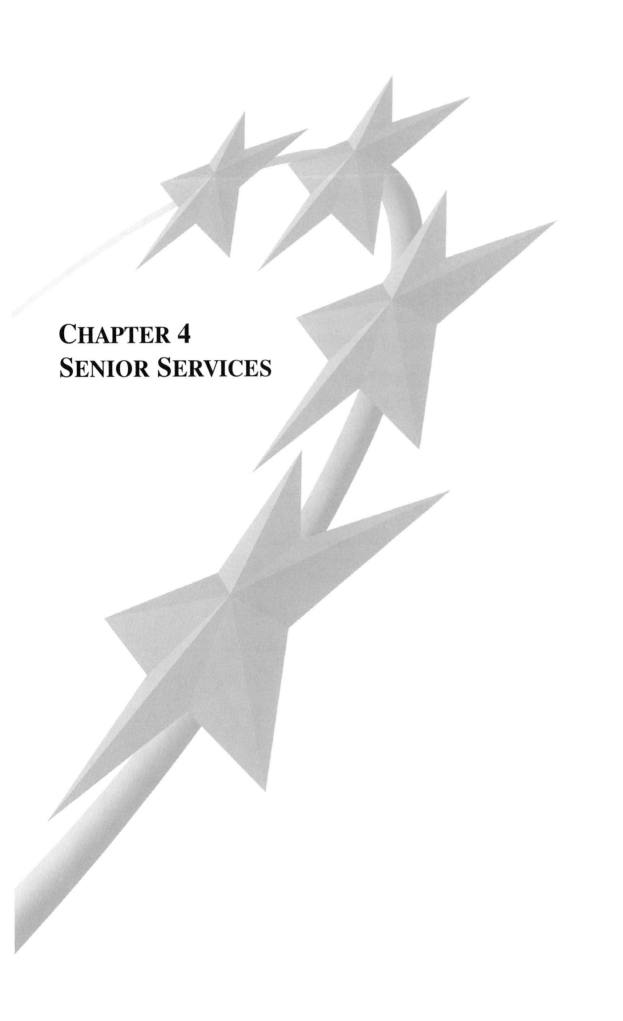

CHAPTER 4
SENIOR SERVICES

SENIOR SERVICES

When Friendly Acres Retirement Community investigated alternative approaches to care that would improve the well-being and quality of life of residents, Snoezelen was discovered. This multisensory therapeutic approach stimulates the senses to induce relaxation. Friendly Acres administers Snoezelen from both white and dark rooms, each of which is designed to produce different effects.

Imagine a room bathed in different colors and with beautiful scenes projected onto the walls, the sounds of soft music and a bubbling brook in the background, the scent of lavender in the air. It is a place to relax and free oneself from worries of the outside world; a place where it is enough just to be, without needing to do anything. This is the concept behind Snoezelen therapy and it is one of several programs Friendly Acres Retirement Community initiated to bring about "culture change" through innovative programming rather than through costly changes to our physical facility.

Originally developed in the Netherlands in the 1970s for use with mentally and physically disabled individuals and geared primarily toward children, Snoezelen—coined from two Dutch words meaning "to sniff 'and "to doze" —is a philosophy of care involving the stimulation of all five senses that is now recognized for its benefits in geriatric care. A Snoezelen environment encourages trust and relaxation, and it is designed to stimulate the senses without the need for intellectual activity. The effects of Snoezelen are many, yet somewhat unpredictable, because every person's reaction is unique. Snoezelen has greatly enhanced the quality of life for many residents by improving mood, memory, relaxation, and socialization.

The Friendly Acres journey into the realm of Snoezelen began in a small closet-sized room where we attempted to predict what kinds of benefits Snoezelen could bring to our community. The results of this test program were promising. Residents who were involved exhibited improved behavior, and we documented a decrease in the need to medicate some of the participants. This encouraged us to explore its use further—not only for the benefit of our own residents but for long term care in general. Our experience has been that multi-sensory therapy appears to be an under-recognized tool in caring for the elderly.

With a $38,000 grant awarded to Friendly Acres by the United Methodist Health Ministry Fund, we set up two rooms that included a variety of multisensory elements including aromatherapy, bubble lights, relaxation music, vibra-massage seating, interactive music with sound beams, tactile boards, and fiber optic lights.

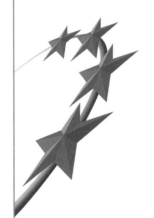

Friendly Acres Retirement Community

Newton, Kan.

To our knowledge, Friendly Acres is the first geriatric facility in the nation to have developed both a "white room" and a "dark room" for Snoezelen interventions. Both settings offer similar treatments but with different techniques. The dark room, with its dark walls and ceilings, introduces ultraviolet lighting. Ultraviolet rays makes colors "pop." It is amazing to see the residents' reactions when observing colors under the black light. One resident whose vision had been impaired from macular degeneration had tears in her eyes exclaiming over the beautiful colors. The bright colors under the black light enabled her to distinguish color with clarity she had not experienced in many years.

A staff attendant documents the resident's exhibited behavior before, during, and after each session and notes which pieces of equipment were used during the session. The School of Nursing at Wichita State University is auditing our documentation of resident use and reactions to determine outcomes, such as reduction in the use of psychotropic medications, improved behavioral issues, and improved socialization skills.

In addition to scheduled sessions, our staff takes residents to the Snoezelen rooms when they display inappropriate behaviors or when it is perceived that multisensory therapy may be an appropriate intervention. For those living in a group environment such as long term care, not only does the participant benefit from his or her time in the Snoezelen environment, but other residents and staff receive secondary benefits from the calming effects it offers. A number of employees use the Snoezelen rooms for relaxation breaks, and some report positive effects of Snoezelen exposure during the onset of migraine headaches.

Friendly Acres is now developing an educational program to help other organizations set up similar programs in their facilities. We are considering making the Snoezelen rooms available for use by residents in the community. The fees we collect for this service will help us fund the expansion of the program.

Multisensory stimulation can deliver benefits to people of all ages and as we have learned from our experiences, Snoezelen is especially successful in restoring dignity and quality of life to the elderly.

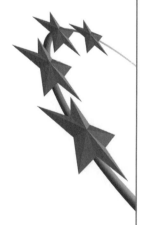

Friendly Acres
Retirement
Community

Newton, Kan.

A stimulating environment for living was created when United Retirement Center became certified as an Eden Alternative facility, partnered with Easter Seals South Dakota to add a child development center on its campus, and collaborated with South Dakota State University to become a training site for students. The residents and day care clients of this community that has skilled nursing, assisted and independent living, and respite care, are surrounded by children, students, staff, and pets. This age-integrated community offers benefits to everyone involved.

Project ALIVE—Alleviating Loneliness in a Vibrant Environment—sustains and enhances our community with employment, education and life. United Retirement Center's (URC) residents, staff, senior day care clients; children enrolled at Easter Seals Child Development Center; and students from South Dakota State University enjoy enhanced living with intergenerational programs. We provide a meaningful environment for living to people 4 weeks to 104 years of age.

URC implemented Project ALIVE to counter the outdated notion that hospitals cure the sick and nursing homes house the dying. Our certification as an Eden Alternative facility created the foundation for our initiative. We ascribe to the Eden Alternative philosophy, which promotes "human habitats for the living" to alleviate three plagues of long term care: loneliness, helplessness, and boredom. At URC, residents are surrounded by animals, including two dogs, six cats, one rabbit, and several birds. Lush plants and bright colors add to our vibrant environment, as do our committed employees who engage our residents in activities and conversation. The full spectrum of our services was enhanced when we affiliated with Easter Seals South Dakota and South Dakota State University (SDSU) to expand our vision. Children now share our living spaces. Students enrolled in the university visit daily.

The Easter Seals Child Development Center (ESCDC) cares for 60 children who participate in a developmentally appropriate atmosphere of daily intergenerational activities and interactions. The center's purpose is to provide quality education and intervention services for children and families in an inclusive age-integrated community.

South Dakota has one of the highest percentages of working mothers in the nation, which places extra challenges on child day care facilities. Fifty percent of the children served by ESCDC are in families of single parents who receive assistance through a federally funded CCAMPIS (Child Care Access Means Parents In School) program. At least a dozen of the children have special needs, or are monitored by the department of Social Services, or have been sent through a community domestic abuse shelter. Individual assessment and screening for all children enrolled in the program helps staff address their needs in a safe, inclusive environment.

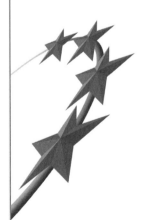

United Retirement Center

Brookings, S.D.

United Retirement Center abides by its mission to provide clients with the highest quality care, recognizing the human dignity of residents while helping them achieve physical, social, and emotional balance. Such efforts are achieved through the caring for our animals and tending to gardens by planting and harvesting crops. Activities with children in the ESCDC offer immeasurable opportunities for interactions on field trips, as well as daily communication with youngsters.

Intergenerational activities are coordinated by professional staff cross-trained to serve clients on both ends of the age continuum. Full-time ESCDC staff must complete 20 hours of training each year in areas such as child growth and development, and they plan learning activities and communicate with the families.

The third component in this community effort involves our connection with SDSU. For students who take courses in early childhood development or nursing, through SDSU's Family and Consumer Sciences programs, it is a perfect fit. Students rotate through our facilities, doing academic assignments while gaining practical experience. Students enrolled in journalism, pre-veterinary, engineering, and pharmacy programs have also completed assignments on our campus.

Due to parents working to support their families, childcare issues are of utmost importance to families in South Dakota. The excellent childcare services that are provided on the URC campus have met important needs experienced by community residents, as well as URC staff. As a national crisis lingers for licensed nurses and certified nurse aides, URC has one of the lowest employee turnover rates in the nation. We believe the close proximity that our staff is able to maintain to their children at the ESCDC is a contributing factor in employee retention.

United Retirement Center remains committed to enhancing resident and staff satisfaction and developing a vibrant environment in which six generations can grow and thrive. We are proud that human beings whose ages span more than 100 years are served and nourished by this loving community.

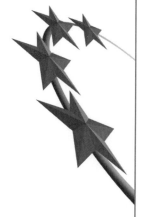

United Retirement Center

Brookings, S.D.

Although restraints are commonly used by long term care providers to reduce the risk of falls, there is no evidence that restraints prevent falls or injuries. Windy Hill Village of the Presbyterian Homes launched the Kaleidoscope Initiative℠ as a resident-centered care philosophy with the goal of becoming restraint-free. Through collaboration with the Pennsylvania Restraint Reduction Initiative, Windy Hill Village eliminated the use of physical restraints. Achieving this goal fueled commitment to develop similar resident-centered approaches to performance improvement and service delivery.

Windy Hill Village was in the 38th percentile among long term care providers in the Commonwealth of Pennsylvania for use of physical restraints. We formed a restraint reduction team when it became evident that restraint use was, in fact, not in the best interests of our residents. To the contrary, studies show that residents who are restrained have the potential for physical and mental decline. Initially the team was led by the administrator and the director of nursing, with nursing supervisors, licensed practical nurses, nursing assistants, activities staff, social workers, and therapists participating as members. The team struggled in the beginning to accept the rationale for the restraint reduction plan. The members were sure that they were making sound decisions and that the restraints kept their residents "safe." It was obvious that education would be one of the key ingredients for restraint reduction.

The team called the Pennsylvania Restraint Reduction Initiative (PARRI) for consultation. PARRI is dedicated to reducing restraints by providing education and support to long term care facilities that are willing to make this commitment to excellence in care. Members of our team attended a seminar, which described situations and showed pictures of residents who had been seriously injured or died as the result of restraint use. Following this presentation, they returned to the facility with a burning passion to eliminate the use of restraints.

This marked the birth of our initiative. The desire to reduce restraints no longer had anything to do with quality indicator measurements but rather, a sincere commitment to assure that the rights of the residents were protected and that quality of life was improved. It was a turning point for the staff. Team meetings were revamped, and the process for restraint reduction took on a whole new life.

As part of any transforming process, the mindset for change is intangible but key to success. The challenge to educate all staff members, families, therapists, and physicians seemed at times to be overwhelming. The team set out to reduce the use of physical restraints in a slow methodical way. Each nursing unit was to reduce one restraint at a time. The process involved

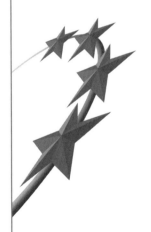

Windy Hill Village

Philipsburg, Pa.

all departments within the facility. At in-service classes, the team members reenacted some of the drawings they had seen by using a mannequin to depict a resident falling to the floor or hanging in a side rail. Employees attending in-service trainings were restrained for the entire hour so they could experience what residents would experience in a similar situation. The resulting indignation was contagious. The right questions were being asked, and decisions were made proactively.

We established a restraint-free policy, and within a year, we were ranked in the 2nd percentile. Within several years, we were completely restraint-free. Celebrating success was important to the process. Each time a restraint was removed, it was more than a number being removed from the logs. It meant the resident's needs had been thoroughly reviewed, preferences identified, routines known, pain managed, environments customized, restorative programs developed, and more personalized care added. It meant that every day could be a "best day" for our residents.

Financial support was supplied by Presbyterian Homes for equipment and supplies such as low beds, dense mats, customized wheelchairs and chairs sized to fit the individuals, devices to prevent wheelchairs from moving when the resident stands, non-skid slippers, defined perimeter mattresses with beveled edges, body pillows, and pressure-reducing seat cushions.

Throughout the process, the team monitored the fall rate and degree of injuries related to falls. The team found that with the restraint elimination program, the number of falls remained the same, but the severity of the injuries decreased dramatically.

The success of restraint elimination became a cornerstone for culture change in our facility. The Restraint Reduction Team was renamed the "Vision Team," and we envisioned ways to become more resident-focused. We no longer develop care plans in a conference room. We meet in the resident's room, where the resident and caregivers—family members; the primary nursing assistant; the RN supervisor; social services, activities, chaplain, dietitian, and restorative staff assemble. The meeting is more like a gathering of friends visiting a person they care very much about. While in the resident's room, the care plan comes alive because everyone interacts with the resident within his or her environment. The most frequently asked question is, "How can we help you have your best day?" The residents' replies have ranged from "I'd like someone to read the paper to me," to "Tonight, I want to soak for a half-hour when I get my bath."

Delivery systems have changed as well. We offer numerous dining times, select menus, and restorative programs each day. We have made many changes because throughout our care center, we assure safety and deliver service without restraint.

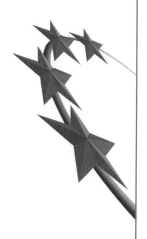

Windy Hill Village

Philipsburg, Pa.

98

Therapeutic cooking is one way some nursing home residents cope with medical, emotional, and social disabilities. The Chef's Club is a monthly program that engages Long Island State Veterans Home residents in planning and preparing a gourmet meal. Chef's Club offers residents a sense of community and autonomy and enables them to continue participating in an activity they may have enjoyed in the past.

The Long Island State Veterans Home has emerged as one of our region's premiere providers of long term skilled nursing service and medical adult day care. Located on the State University of New York at Stony Brook campus, we operate 350 inpatient beds and provide adult day care to 50 outpatients. The Long Island State Veterans Home remains one of the only nursing homes in the country that is fully integrated into the health and educational missions of a major teaching and research university. It is with enthusiasm for this mission that each of our more than 500 employees strives each day to maintain a world-class health care facility for America's heroes and provide a place that aging veterans will always be able to call home.

In keeping with this vital mission, the Veterans Home staff has embarked on many progressive initiatives designed to enhance each resident's overall experience. One of these programs is the Chef's Club, a gourmet meal preparation program for 25 to 30 veteran residents. This program gives our residents opportunities to engage in a creative process with their peers. Quality of life is increased while helping individuals sustain cognition, physical mobility, and psycho/social health.

Residents are referred to the program by members of an interdisciplinary treatment team. For example, someone from nutritional services may be concerned that a resident is losing weight and not eating. A social worker may identify tendencies of self-isolation among individuals who led active lives before coming into the nursing home. Nursing staff may recognize individuals whose activities of daily living are decreasing due to lack of physical activity. A recreation therapist may learn that an individual enjoys cooking. All team members can refer residents who may benefit from this program. Participation in the Chef's Club can be a good way to meet a resident's leisure needs and help him or her adjust to the facility and maintain active socialization.

The Chef's Club program has evolved into a democratic process with rules and standards devised by the participants. The residents must be medically stable, able to feed themselves, and have limited dietary restrictions. All participants attend a planning meeting during which the menu is devised and voted upon. A typical menu consists of shrimp cocktail, tossed salad, corn on the cob, garlic bread, steak or chicken, and pie á la mode for dessert.

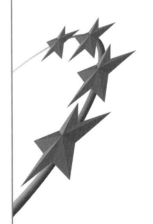

Long Island State Veterans Home
Stony Brook, N.Y.

Once the menu is decided, it is submitted to the food service department so the food can be ordered. The meal preparation begins around 4 p.m. Residents cut vegetables and fruits; make sauces, dressings, hors d'oeuvres, and bread; and set the tables. The clinical staff does the actual cooking and grilling. There is a strong emphasis on maintaining safety and observing food preparation precautions. After eating the home cooked meal the residents assist with cleaning up.

Residents in nursing homes often complain of being served institutional food. Chef's Club provides the opportunity to eat food similar to what was prepared at home and helps to increase resident satisfaction, happiness, and well-being. The success of this program is evidenced by the many years it has run and the consistent attendance participants at the meal planning and preparation sessions. The program has also been validated by verbal comments of satisfaction. Chef's Club has not only heightened self-esteem, but has also helped to build community. It is a program that serves the needs of a very special population, "America's heroes."

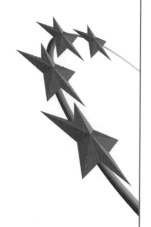

Long Island State Veterans Home
Stony Brook, N.Y.

Smart service providers are constantly asking, "How can we better meet the needs of our customers?" When the answer is a valued service that provides a new stream of income, it is a win-win for both parties. Rockwood's Gourmet Chef on Wheels program was inaugurated to provide more than 200 residents of a retirement community the opportunity to enjoy catered epicurean meals in their own homes. The gourmet meal program is valued by the residents, and it has produced revenue in excess of $12,000 annually.

Gourmet Chef on Wheels provides quality, gourmet meals to the independent living residents of Rockwood Forest Estates, an upscale retirement neighborhood of single-family residences and duplexes on the campus of Rockwood South, a facility of Rockwood Retirement Communities. Located on an 80-acre woodland in Spokane, Wash., more than 200 residents live in Rockwood Forest Estates.

Residents wanted a reliable source of excellent meals that could be delivered to their homes if they were ill, did not wish to cook, or were entertaining friends or family. The solution to meet this need came from the ingenuity of the staff of the food service department. The Gourmet Chef on Wheels service began with just a few special-occasion meals delivered to residents, and it has grown into a profitable monthly service that provides value to the residents.

Residents choose their entrée(s), side dishes, and beverages from a menu that is circulated throughout the community. The dates of availability of menu items are noted in the residents' in-house newsletter and advertised in promotional mail. Orders are taken by phone, fax, and over the Rockwood computer network to make it easy for residents to participate. Meals are packaged, labeled with instructions, and delivered by our general manager and the gourmet chef using the Gourmet Chef on Wheels golf cart. This allows for greater interaction between Rockwood Forest Estates residents and our personnel, and it helps us stay close to our customers.

Marketing efforts have been important, and have included the creation of a unique logo for Gourmet Chef on Wheels, gift certificates, comment cards, brochures, and the menus with special themes.

Gourmet Chef on Wheels has proved to fill a need for the residents of Rockwood Forest Estates, enabling them to live in their independent environment longer, enjoy a higher quality of life, maintain good nutrition, and entertain family and friends in style, without the time and effort of cooking.

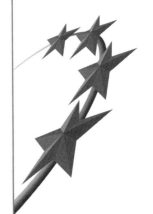

Rockwood Retirement Community

Spokane, Wash.

Resident satisfaction in long term care is often an issue of control. When routines are interrupted or traditions are changed, it can be disorienting and upsetting to residents. When Eger Health Care and Rehabilitation Center initiated improvements in response to resident feedback, the staff discovered that changes in residents' dining and meal service must be accomplished slowly.

Members of food services, nursing, social services, and administration at Eger Health Care and Rehabilitation Center interviewed residents and family members and then discussed ways to improve residents' satisfaction with meals and related food services. Findings were discussed with team members and plans of action were formulated to improve and exceed resident and family expectations. Our primary finding, resulting from experience rather than this initial research, was to go slowly. Introduction of new menu items, changes in staff, reordering of tray deliveries, or computerization of menus are actually perceived as major interruptions and threaten control.

Despite persistent complaints about food, once a new menu and delivery system were introduced, many residents longed for the old system. As a result, we had to backpedal and slow down our introduction of new and innovative foods and services.

What we all learned was that change is difficult, but not impossible. Changes must be made in pencil. Erasers are necessary and serve as useful tools in the change process. Residents and families can teach us many things. Personal, repetitive interactions with families provide the best advantage for eventual change. If families and residents understand the rationale for change and are kept apprised of the status of changes, accommodation of change evolves.

Long term care is very different from acute care. Each long term care facility has its own culture and its own ability to adjust to changes, especially with food. Staff is no different. Employees exhibit tolerance of and desire for change at varying rates. Perception is reality. Understanding this fact makes change easier.

We knew that modifications to our meal services were necessary to meet the needs of a more culturally and demographically diverse population of residents. Despite the fact that we moved more slowly than we anticipated, we were ultimately able to achieve our objectives.

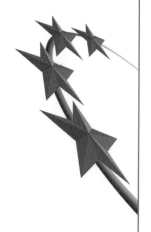

Eger
Health Care

Staten Island, N.Y.

Creating a positive dining experience for residents demands more than white tablecloths and thicker sauces; it requires a change in mindset. To give residents more choice and control, Westchester Care Center created a restaurant-like atmosphere and services, but not before examining attitudes about dining and reorienting staff to think differently about meal service and the needs experienced by residents.

Westchester Care Center emphasizes to staff that the ability to make choices is important to resident well-being. Choices give a resident the feeling of control and alleviate, to some degree, the feeling of loss that occurs when one is admitted to a care center.

On examination we found that mealtime was not a great source of pleasure and that an attitude of "feeding" prevailed. One of our first steps was to eliminate the word "feeding" when it came to meal times in the dining room. Cows and chickens are fed, not people. The concept of "dining," in contrast to "feeding," became our main focus. We needed to create a restaurant atmosphere. We decided to set the tables in the main dining room with placemats for breakfast and supper and use tablecloths and cloth napkins for the noon meal. Silverware is placed, as are glasses and cups. The menu is posted daily on a board just outside the dining room. Music or some type of entertainment is provided during the mid-day dining experience.

When the residents are seated, the wait staff prepares two plates, each with the featured entrées of the day. These are presented so residents may look at the food and choose which items they wish to have for their meal. The meal is then plated and served to them, rather than being placed before them on a tray. The wait staff pours beverages and assists residents with buttering bread and handling other condiments. Medication carts are never brought into the dining room. If meds are given at mealtime, they are presented in a cup, brought into the dining room by the nurse. Efforts are made to seat residents with other residents with whom they are compatible. Those residents who require assistance receive their meals in smaller rooms where they can receive one-on-one attention.

The dietary department is proud of its contribution to improve the lives of residents. We take pride in the reputation of the department, and each of us strives to maintain our reputation of making life better for our residents.

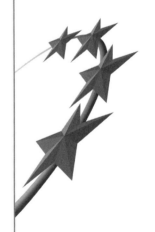

Westchester Care Center

Tempe, Ariz.

Neshaminy Manor wanted to provide residents with a dining experience celebrating the '50s era. The goal was to provide a reminiscent environment, which was supported by individual choices in foods, and thus, the New York Deli was born. As part of their daily activities, residents made decorations, such as music notes and records (LPs) that were hung from the ceiling in the room where the deli was to be located.

When Neshaminy Manor decided to create the New York Deli, we knew that it would be important to include residents in the planning. They responded with enthusiasm.

The activities, dietary, nursing, and admissions departments, residents and volunteers all worked together in a collaborative effort to produce the New York Deli. The residents of one nursing unit made homemade bread loaves, which they varnished and displayed in a basket, with jars of peppers, olives, and artichoke hearts. A volunteer constructed a full-size deli counter. The glass front provided residents with a view of luncheon meats, cheeses, bread, coleslaw, and all the trimmings. The activities department also built a '50s style jukebox.

The waitresses wore black poodle skirts, white shirts with pink scarves, and waiters wore black pants with white shirts. As residents visited the New York Deli, they ordered corned beef, turkey club, or any combination of sandwich preferences offered. All of these food choices were offered in therapeutic diet form, puree, ground, renal, thickened liquids or lactose free. Residents selected New York egg cream or root beer as the beverages of the day.

Over six weeks, each of the 60-bed nursing units had an opportunity to experience the New York Deli. The smiles and discussion about the initiative proves that dining events enriched the experiences of the residents at Neshaminy Manor.

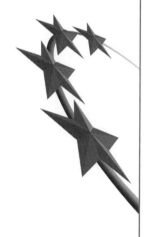

Neshaminy Manor

Warrington, Pa.

One way to respond to complaints is to involve customers in solutions to address dissatisfaction. When Providence Mount St. Vincent discovered that residents were not satisfied with food service, residents were asked to participate on the committee that was formed to address their concerns. Meal service events were one area where improvements were needed.

Even after the completion of a major renovation of the main kitchen and dining areas, Providence Mount St. Vincent continued to receive resident complaints about food. This reaction was a surprise because we had introduced a select menu and a new dining option with wait staff service. In response, a Resident Participation Committee, made up of residents and food service staff, was formed to address concerns about food service. Based on the feedback, the food service department planned a schedule of theme-oriented meal service events.

At least once each menu cycle, we create a special menu to introduce more variety into what we offer. We establish a theme and plan menu selections, decorations, and entertainment accordingly. The menu for our summer solstice party in June included marinated flank steak and barbecued chicken. Tables were decorated with a summer theme, and special music was provided in both the café and dining room.

While Seattle was hosting the All-Star game in July, it was a perfect time for an All-Star celebration. "Stadium" menu selections were offered for lunch and dinner. Rooms were decorated with baseball memorabilia and trivia. Baseball movies, including, *"Pride of the Yankees"* and *"It Happens Every Spring"* were featured in the café and popcorn was served.

Dining areas were decorated with a Hawaiian theme in August for our luau event. Flower leis were presented to each resident. Luncheon and dinner menus featured Pacific cuisine. Live entertainment was provided by one of our employees, who, after sharing Hawaiian history and customs, did hula dances and then instructed residents how to hula.

Every summer, Providence Mount St. Vincent hosts a summer concert series. Held in the evenings on the patio, this year's entertainment included Big Band, Jazz, Country Western, and Brazilian music. The food service team wrote special menus for each night to complement the musical theme. Future events include an Oktoberfest celebration in September and a Halloween party in October. We will add a monthly brunch to bring more families together to dine with residents. We also will feature a resident recipe each month that is woven into the menu. The active participation of residents is good and reinforces the value of customer feedback. As a result of these events and other changes we have made based on resident feedback, we are pleased that compliments are replacing complaints.

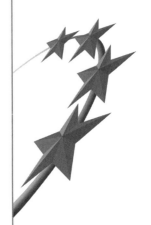

*Providence
Mount St. Vincent*

Seattle, Wash.

Alzheimer's disease and related dementia have become the fourth leading causes of death among older adults. Despite the size of this special-needs population, estimated at around 480,000 nationwide, nutritional approaches have not been widely instituted. After identifying troubling weight loss in advanced dementia residents, Glencroft Care Center developed and perfected nutritional approaches to improve the care and comfort of residents with this disease.

According to the Arizona Alzheimer's Association, "persons with advanced dementia are poorly understood and marginally cared for...a special high-needs population that has historically received nominal custodial care and very little attention or recognition." After identifying significant weight loss in 28% of Glencroft Care Center's residents with diagnosis of advanced dementia, we redesigned our nutritional approaches.

Determining that a possible cause of weight loss in advanced dementia is due to a resident's inability to consume adequate calories through traditional meal and snack programs, we implemented three programs: Contemporary Cuisine, the Innovative Dining Environment Approach (IDEA), and Supplemental Snacks-Shakes. The Contemporary Cuisine program aimed to improve the quality of pureed food, while the IDEA improved feeding techniques. The Supplemental Snacks-Shakes program consisted of a seven-day snack rotation, and was made available to residents 24 hours a day.

Patients in Glencroft's special care unit for persons with advanced dementia, known as the Purple Sage Unit, benefited from these initiatives. The combination of these programs resulted in a dramatic reduction of weight loss over a 6-month period. A grant-funded partnership between Glencroft and the Arizona Alzheimer's Association made this program financially possible. Staff from nursing, dietary, activities, social services, as well as the chaplain and administrative personnel were involved.

Within six months of instituting these programs, the percentage of significant weight loss for residents in the Purple Sage Unit decreased to 5% and it represented a 23% reduction over this short period of time. This initiative earned Glencroft Care Center a best practice award from the Arizona Association of Homes and Housing for the Aging. The Purple Sage Unit was recognized for "defining and articulating programs and care-giving methods that promote the comfort, dignity, and quality of life of its residents."

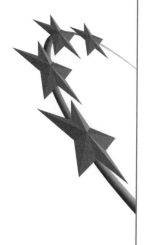

Glencroft Care Center

Glendale, Ariz.

Studies show that moving is a very stressful event in one's life. This is particularly true for a person who is facing relocation from a home, where they have lived independently, into a residential care facility. It is also true for a person who is moving from one section of a continuing care community to another. La Posada at Park Centre approaches these transitions with compassion and thoughtful attention to the needs of all who are affected by the move.

On the La Posada at Park Centre campus, a Settling In Team is available to help residents move to another level of care or to welcome new residents of our community.

Recognizing that it is often traumatic for a resident to transfer from independent living to assisted living or from assisted living to a nursing home, the Settling In Team is available to visit with the residents, discuss which items of furniture are most important to them, measure new spaces to determine where and how the resident's possessions will be accommodated, arrange for movers, and ship items that will not be moved to family members. We often hear, "I'm not ready yet" when residents are anticipating a move. Residents who do not have children or relatives to assist them feel especially overwhelmed. The Settling In Team can do everything from simple hand-holding to full move-in coordination, including hanging pictures on the walls and unpacking boxes.

The Settling In Team has made a positive difference in La Posada's ability to meet the needs of current and incoming residents in a professional and caring way. The team members are compassionate, caring, and patient. They possess good organization and communication skills. The team's keen sense of interior decorating comes into play as well. Their work involves a quiet demeanor of support to ensure that the dignity, independence, and choices of the residents are honored.

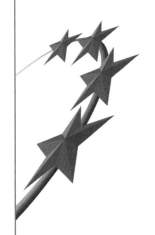

La Posada at Park Centre

Green Valley, Ariz.

First impressions form lasting impressions and that's why Jupiter Medical Center warmly welcomes new residents to its sub-acute and long term care pavilion. This hospitality helps to bridge the transition and forms a solid foundation on which to build a satisfying experience.

The Shining Star Program was implemented in response to the emotional needs of individuals who are admitted to Jupiter Medical Center Pavilion's 120-bed, sub-acute rehabilitation and long term care facility. The purpose of this program is to warmly welcome each new resident and to become a friendly face they can count on.

Before a new patient or resident is admitted, a gold Mylar star balloon anchored with a beautiful card is placed in the resident's room. The card features a poem written by a Pavilion staff member, welcoming the new resident to the facility. Shortly after admission, a designated Shining Star representative visits the new resident and continues to visit throughout the duration of his or her stay. During these visits, any comments or concerns are directed to department managers via a Star Communication Form, expediting the process for service recovery. If and when the guest returns home, the Shining Star sends a handwritten note to the guest's home to thank him or her for the privilege of providing service.

All Shining Stars project a positive attitude and reassure new patients that a caring, responsive team of professionals will care for and about them. Each Shining Star extends a commitment to make the Pavilion living experience positive and memorable—and contributes to making the Jupiter Medical Center Pavilion stand out as the shining star it is in this community.

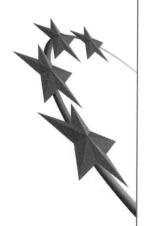

Jupiter Medical Center Pavilion

Jupiter, Fla.

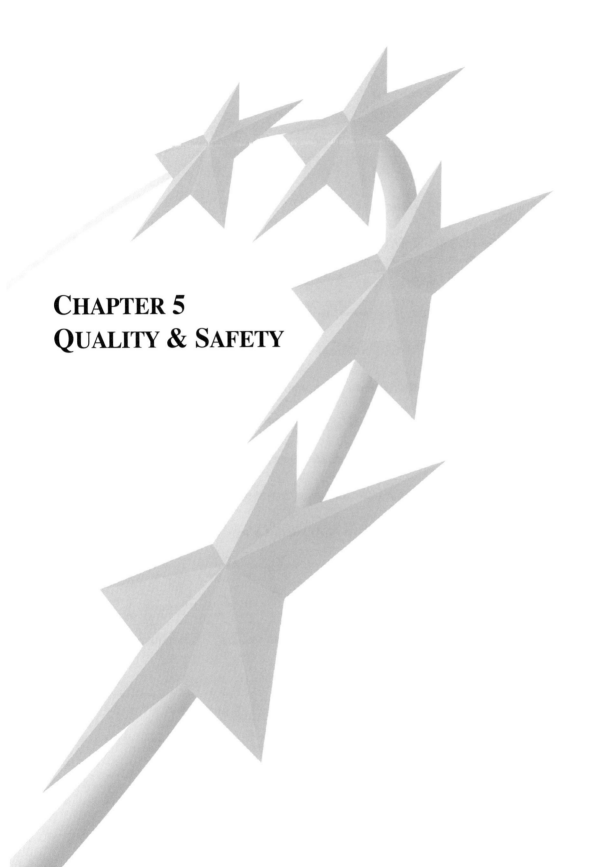

CHAPTER 5
QUALITY & SAFETY

Decisions about where to focus attention and invest resources to improve outcomes of care or operational performance require data. Lacking a reliable structure to analyze data and gauge performance, Daughters of Israel created a Continuous Quality Improvement Committee. The committee reviews and analyzes a range of data on a regular basis and targets improvement opportunities that will benefit the residents of this long term care facility and the clients of the adult day care center. This has enabled the organization to maintain a prioritized list of improvement opportunities based on a more rigorous review of data and committee consensus.

The Continuous Quality Improvement (CQI) program at Daughters of Israel (DOI) is designed to evaluate, maintain, and improve the quality of care and the quality of life for residents in the facility and clients of the Herr Adult Medical Day Center. The organization-wide program strives to ensure that resident and client care are consistent with achievable goals. This is accomplished through a list of reports published by our quality assurance director. The list identifies the data to be collected and the frequency of each collection. The committee meets on a weekly basis and reviews data on employee turnover, resident falls, infection rates, water temperatures, fire and disaster drills, pressure ulcers, restraints, knowledge of emergency procedures, medication administration, employee education, and numerous other related areas.

Opportunities for improvement are identified based on the review of aggregate data from many sources. Some of these areas include analysis of trends and statistics from department reports, subcommittees, performance improvement teams, standing committees, and regulatory agencies. Verbal and/or written concerns from residents, families, and the community are also analyzed. Feedback from administration, department heads, clinical staff, consultants, and employees is solicited. Satisfaction surveys from residents' families and DOI employees are reviewed.

CQI activities are meant to encourage communication and teamwork among all departments. Identified opportunities for improvement are expected to be solved at the level of staff most closely involved with the issue and, where appropriate, in an interdisciplinary format.

The goals and objectives of the CQI Committee include the following: 1) monitor the system for collecting accurate and meaningful information concerning quality issues; 2) review the indicators and statistics that determine quality performance; 3) monitor and evaluate the quality of service and pursue opportunities to improve quality of care, quality of life, and quality of service; 4) identify patterns and trends that could represent potential opportunities for improvement, as well as respond to

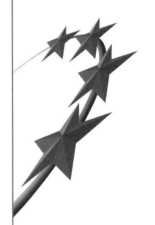

Daughters of Israel

West Orange, N.J.

actual opportunities for improvement as they occur; 5) communicate the goals and results of quality management projects to all "customers" in the process, including residents, clients, families and staff; 6) emphasize the need for involvement of all staff in the activities of a quality improvement program; 7) maintain a prioritized list of opportunities for improvement, based upon aggregate data submitted to the CQI Oversight Committee and data collected and reviewed from all departments; 8) establish Performance Improvement Teams (PIT) to develop a process for improvement related to specific issues; 9) provide facility-wide education on all CQI activities and outcomes through house-wide orientations, department specific orientations and in-services; 10) establish an annual calendar for review of data collections within the facility; and 11) utilize organizational, state, federal, regional, national benchmarks as comparison tools to identify opportunities for improvement.

The CQI oversight committee may also assign specific issues to the facility's care plan teams or to specific departments for resolution. All staff is oriented to current performance improvement activities. All department heads and supervisors are educated in performance improvement. Performance improvement information is disseminated to staff through departmental staff meetings, in-service education, fliers, and storyboards.

PITs are used to design new systems or processes or to improve existing systems or processes for which opportunities for improvement are identified. The teams are interdisciplinary and include members from all involved departments. Department heads appoint PIT members as requested by the CQI oversight committee. Family members or volunteers may be included on teams at the discretion of the committee. PITs use established performance models that encompass tools such as flow charts, cause and effect diagrams, Pareto charts, histograms, and fishbone diagrams.

We establish our internal aggregate data collections and measure our performance improvement over time. Data are benchmarked against the facility, research studies, state and federal data and statistics, and literature. Benchmarks such as quality indicator reports, software vendor reports, and best practices are used. An annual written report is made to the DOI Board of Governors. Storyboards of selected projects are presented to the board at the same time.

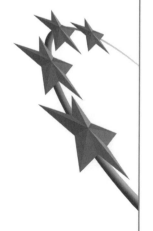

***Daughters
of Israel***

West Orange, N.J.

The Olympic Medical Quality Institute is a forum designed to select and introduce medical quality initiatives at Olympic Medical Center. The institute has effectively engaged medical and community participation in pursuing evidence-based quality improvement, and it has helped prioritize information technology decisions. At monthly public meetings, the Olympic Medical Quality Institute discusses quality improvement initiatives, accomplishments, and future plans.

The Olympic Medical Quality Institute (OMQI) was created to examine quality improvement ideas and to help guide Olympic Medical Center (OMC) in its strategic pursuit of quality initiatives and decisions related to information technology. The idea was to convene medical and hospital staff, administration, and board members who were willing to be vocal quality champions and collaborative change agents.

The OMQI has endorsed the principles of the Institute of Medicine's (IOM) report titled, *"Crossing the Quality Chasm"* and the statement of purpose of the Institute for Healthcare Improvement. These guiding principles have enabled OMQI to more effectively review ongoing quality activities at our hospital.

The Olympic Medical Quality Institute has given local physicians and hospital leaders the opportunity to influence quality and information technology decisions. It has provided a better understanding of the quality transformation, as envisioned by the Institute for Healthcare Improvement.

A quality scorecard was restructured by a subcommittee of OMQI to be organized under the six "aims" identified in the IOM's Chasm report. This scorecard is presented each month at public board meetings. This has led to closer scrutiny of the rationale behind each of the quality initiatives we undertake. OMQI regularly receives updated reports on the status of information technology use and reviews opportunities to move forward in this area. This has provided a more integrated and rational lens for viewing information technology needs.

OMQI provides leadership to the Transforming Health Care in Clallam County project. This project has successfully recruited physicians to work together with patients, agencies, businesses, and community leaders. Its aim is to implement measurable improvement in the quality of local medical care based on evidence of best practices. Another initiative involves balance-exercise classes (with objective measurements of improvement) for the elderly who are at-risk for falls. One task force is coordinating stakeholders among local health care institutions and services to achieve community-wide acceptance of physician-ordered life sustaining treatment orders. An improved pathway for symptomatic breast screening/diagnosis to decrease

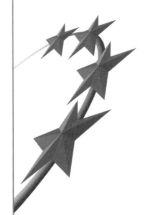

*Olympic
Medical
Center*

Port Angeles, Wash.

and standardize the time for workup has been accomplished. Work is now ongoing with a chemotherapy orders trial and a medication reconciliation project.

The Olympic Medical Quality Institute is a successful forum for carefully reviewing options for medical quality and information technology improvements at Olympic Medical Center. It has been effective in catalyzing the involvement of various provider and community constituencies in our efforts to improve health care quality.

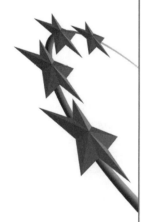

*Olympic
Medical
Center*

Port Angeles, Wash.

Benchmarking is a valuable tool that enables institutions to compare processes and outcomes with similar institutions. Gibson General Hospital discovered that there were no comparable, affordable databases to meet to meet the benchmarking needs of rural health care providers. In light of this unmet need, they formed a company dedicated specifically to meet quality improvement needs of the rural health care industry. Each month, more than 90 participating organizations submit data. Gibson General collects, aggregates, and returns data to participants in a benchmark report. The rural providers are then able to use the data to identify best practices, exchange information, and conduct quality improvement reviews of their facilities.

During the annual review of Gibson General Hospital's quality improvement program, we identified the need to benchmark our processes with other rural facilities. This began a search for a program that would meet our needs. A thorough review of the programs offered nationally revealed nothing that would meet our needs as a rural health care provider. The available programs were primarily focused on processes unique to tertiary facilities. The costs were prohibitive for a rural facility struggling to survive in the era of managed health care.

With these findings in mind, the performance improvement director of our facility put together a program called "Apples to Apples," which was specific to the needs of rural health care organizations. The first priority was to identify processes that impacted the quality of care delivered to customers that were unique to these organizations. Through networking with rural hospitals in the surrounding area, these processes were identified. Once identified, the remainder of the program was structured. We took into consideration the level of technology available in these facilities, and the amount of time/ personnel that would be needed to facilitate collection of the data. The fees were structured to minimize the impact to the participant's budget, while funding the program to function appropriately.

Each organization is required to collect the requested data on a monthly basis. These data are entered into a database and aggregated with all other reporting facilities. On a quarterly basis, this information is returned to the participating organizations. Each reporting facility receives a report that shows their individual hospital trending, both in narrative form and as a control chart. They also receive an aggregate report, which allows them to compare their processes to every other facility in the program. Through these aggregate reports they are able to identify best practices and exchange information that enables them to improve their own processes and outcomes. Quarterly user group meetings are held to give participating organizations the opportunity to network with other facilities and share information and ideas.

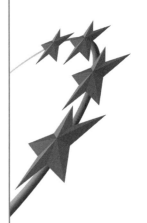

Gibson
General
Hospital

Trenton, Tenn.

During the years we have seen our customers "come of age" technologically. Therefore, we have moved to an Internet-based reporting system. This is having a positive impact because it takes fewer personnel to compile and transmit data to our system. We believe it is having a positive impact on the quality of service we provide.

We have made this program affordable to the end user and have managed to control our overhead costs. This has resulted in a positive financial contribution to our facility. We continue to work to improve the quality of the service that we provide to our customers and to respond to their needs. Many of our customers have long term care facilities and home care services associated with their hospitals. We have now added these classifications to the program.

Rural facilities do not have, for the most part, high-end technology at their beck and call. The only requirements for participation are a computer and Internet access. The simplicity of the program has made it popular. Because of the way it is structured, special training is not required. Participating organizations receive a user manual and can call our performance improvement director if they have any questions.

To develop the Apples to Apples program, we purchased a couple of computer programs and the time of a programmer. We also incurred the costs of applying to the Joint Commission on Accreditation of Healthcare Organizations to be licensed as an ORYX vendor and producing one mailing to hospitals nation-wide. No additional personnel was initially hired to maintain the program, although we recently added a programmer to the staff. The program now has more than 90 participating members nationally.

We conduct annual customer satisfaction surveys and encourage suggestions for improvement. These surveys have been extremely positive and have given us ideas that have helped to improve the services we provide.

The Apples to Apples program has evolved into a national business. A commitment to quality and service drives our delivery and growth. With that in mind, we continue to strive to meet the needs of all who benefit from our services; the participating health care facilities and the customers they serve.

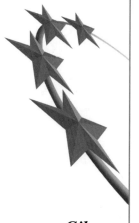

Gibson
General
Hospital

Trenton, Tenn.

The proven Six Sigma methodology is a systematic, data-driven application that focuses on reducing errors to improve quality. This quality improvement strategy has been responsible for streamlining processes and saving billions of dollars for companies like Motorola and General Electric. To improve patient safety and operational efficiency, Froedtert Hospital determined that Six Sigma would be a powerful tool to identify, quantify, and control complex, error-prone hospital processes. The medication administration and laboratory projects described in this profile showed statistically-significant improvements and the outcomes exceeded expectations.

Following publication of the Institute of Medicine's *Quality Chasm* report, Froedtert Hospital formed a consortium that included the American Society for Quality (ASQ), the Medical College of Wisconsin, and CartaNova, a company formed to develop technologies to improve patient safety. This consortium helped to identify Six Sigma projects within our hospital. In determining the selection of projects, we considered sentinel event publications disseminated by the Joint Commission on Accreditation of Healthcare Organizations and medication safety alerts issued by the Institute for Safe Medication Practices. We also considered opportunities for improvement that were identified internally and the interests of various practitioners. Froedtert leaders believed the project would be successful because they embraced the philosophic foundation of Six Sigma that suggests errors do not arise from careless people but from faulty processes.

After prioritizing projects, Froedtert decided to focus initially on: 1) continuous IV infusions, where variation has the potential of causing error, and 2) the collection and handling of laboratory samples, where delays and missing specimens could impact clinical decisions. Both of these projects were complex and involved numerous steps and various departments.

Before projects could be started, we selected and trained employees for "Black Belt" and "Green Belt" facilitation roles. Froedtert and ASQ trained two Black Belts, one Champion, and numerous members of the executive administration team; the first Black Belts included a pharmacist and a nurse. These representatives were selected because they had the extensive experience and skills that are required to be a Black Belt. These include strong communication, project management, leadership, and interpersonal skills. Extensive training in Six Sigma methodology, data collection and statistical analysis is required to become a Six Sigma Black Belt. Froedtert selected a program that required one week of intensive training per month for four months. Concurrent with the four months of training, participants implemented a project to put into practice what they were learning. The director of quality management served as the project champion.

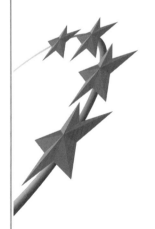

Froedtert Hospital

Milwaukee, Wis.

Dose discrepancy between what the physician orders and what the patient receives has potential to cause great harm to a patient. We found that the lack of standardization in many steps of the process posed a risk for system failure. A high degree of variability was identified in the following steps: 1) MD ordering practices, 2) pharmacy preparation of the IV infusions, 3) RN rate calculation, and 4) RN documentation of IV infusions. A multidisciplinary task force determined standards to reduce variation, and thereby decrease the risk of error. Specific interventions included: 1) establishing standard concentrations for preparation of IV infusions, 2) using a colored label when a nonstandard concentration was necessary, and 3) using a titration table to simplify the rate calculation by the nurse. A "design of experiments" was conducted to assess the impact of each variable on the potential outcome. A determination was made that standardization of IV preparation and use of titration tables to assist in rate calculation had the greatest impact on preventing errors. Thirty days after implementation, measurable improvement was evident. Level 2 discrepancies (defined as a 1-5 mL/hour difference between MD order and actual infusion rate) fell from 21.1% to 11.8%. Level 3 discrepancies (defined as > 5mL/hour difference between MD order and actual infusion rate) fell from 15.8% to 2.9%. These improvements were statistically significant.

Another goal was to decrease the complexity of the current lab processes and improve the cycle, also known as turn-around time. The lab process was defined as "the point a lab order is written or initiated until the results are reported." Every step of this process was studied in detail. One of Six Sigma's tools, "Failure Mode & Effects Analysis" (FMEA), helped prioritize problem areas. The tool assigns points for: 1) likelihood that an error will occur, 2) projected severity of an error if it was to occur, and 3) likelihood that an error would be detected in the current process. FMEA showed that the largest number of errors occurred in the order entry process. Also high on the priority list were errors occurring during specimen collection and inefficiencies of the tube system.

Six Sigma projects showed not only statistically significant improvements, but improvements that superceded expectations. Among the results were: 1) average turnaround time for lab tests ordered STAT fell from 52.7 minutes to 23.1 minutes, 2) timeliness of morning lab draws improved by 150%, 3) pneumatic tube system performance improved with a 25% reduction in average wait times/transactions, and a 73% increase in number of transactions a day.

Six Sigma has helped us reduce patient falls by 43% per 1,000 patient days, decrease patient-controlled analgesic pump programming errors by 56%, and eliminate episodes of life-threatening hypoglycemia associated with insulin therapy without creating hyperglycemia on a surgical intensive care unit. Our improvement continues as we use the tools and training this important initiative introduced.

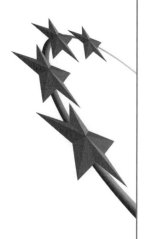

Froedtert
Hospital

Milwaukee, Wis.

St. Mary Medical Center created a Performance Improvement Team to review its special precautions medication process. The opportunity to improve patient safety and reduce the possibility of human error during medication administration was addressed by building visual and tactile cues to easily identify special precaution medications. The plan also called for duplicate checking of these drugs by two nurses and continuous monitoring. After a series of education interventions with nursing staff, compliance with the new process increased from 50% to 100%.

The creation of the special precautions medication process was the result of a request made by staff nurses after a tragic medication error at an area hospital that resulted in the death of a patient. After the incident was reported on the front page of local papers, several nurses approached the quality improvement department and requested that the special precautions medication process be reviewed by a performance improvement team. The nurses were concerned that without prospective review, a similar medication error could happen at St. Mary Medical Center. This represented a consequence that we wanted to avoid at all costs.

A "Failure Mode & Effects Analysis" was performed to identify opportunities to improve the special precautions medication process. The team focused on building a process that would assist the nurse in quickly and accurately identifying that a special precautions medication was being administered through use of tactile, visual, and written stimuli. Bright yellow labels with the words "Special Precautions Medication" were affixed to intravenous fluid bags, forcing nurses to remove the label from the spiking port. The requirement to remove the label signaled a warning to the nurse to slow down and check the patient and drug identification label. Concomitantly, a policy was put into place that required two nurses to verify, initiate, and document use of special precautions medications.

To implement the two initiatives, the team created new nursing guidelines and educated current pharmacy and nursing staff about expectations for the administration of these drugs. Both general and unit orientations of new pharmacy and nursing staff address the process regarding administration of special precautions medications. Questions were added to the nurse's annual review to remind the nurse of the responsibilities and expectations when administering these drugs.

The educational process was non-punitive and focused on re-educating and clarifying responsibilities and expectations. The team studied compliance with the new process for several weeks and found that nurses were in compliance only 50% of the time. Repeat education was performed. Compliance of pharmacy and nursing units is now maintained at 100%.

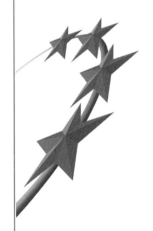

St. Mary Medical Center

Hobart, Ind.

The team addressed the need to continuously monitor performance. Each department that dispenses or administers special precautions medications submits a quality indicator report about compliance. The unit's quality results are posted on the quality bulletin board. Special precaution intravenous bags are randomly sampled to assure the yellow label is affixed to the spiking port. Any deviations from the process are swiftly identified and corrective actions are undertaken.

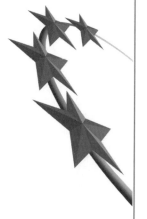

St. Mary
Medical
Center

Hobart, Ind.

Medication errors are the result of failures occurring in the complex processes of prescribing, distributing, administering and monitoring medications. Covenant Healthcare used a Medication Error Reduction Committee to review these processes and implement measures to reduce errors and injuries to patients throughout its system of hospitals and provider sites. Through the program, Covenant Healthcare eliminated verbal orders for high risk medications, educated nurses and physicians, and improved prescription processes.

A Medication Error Reduction Committee (MERC) was formed at Covenant Healthcare as a multidisciplinary, system-wide team charged with reviewing Covenant's medication use process, identifying areas where the safeguards fail, and recommending immediate short and long term measures to reduce the likelihood of medication errors. Site-specific medication safety teams also were formed to implement and monitor process changes at each of Covenant's four hospitals. The committee reported all cross-site recommendations to the Covenant Quality Council for approval. Each medication safety team was responsible for gaining approval for cross-site and site-specific recommendations at its own hospital's Quality Council, implementing the recommendations, and monitoring outcomes. Moreover, they developed educational programs for each initiative and communicated all outcomes to their medical, nursing, and pharmacy staffs.

Utilizing the Medication Safety Self-Assessment instrument from the Institute of Safe Medical Practices (ISMP), which consists of 194 detailed measurements, a review was completed using the multidisciplinary teams from each hospital. The data were then compiled and a single assessment was sent to ISMP for tabulation. The results of the assessment served as the starting point for identifying specific areas on which to focus medication safety efforts.

Over the next year, the MERC and the site-specific Medication Safety Teams (MST) identified areas in the medication use process where failures could occur and developed action plans to address them. The following projects were implemented:

Education. Educating leaders and staff throughout the Covenant System was an important goal of this initiative. The MERC/site-specific MST model was extremely effective as a means of educating core groups on medication errors and disseminating information throughout the entire system.

Verbal Orders for High-Risk Drugs. A system-wide policy was developed that called for written physician orders for such high-risk drugs as chemotherapy

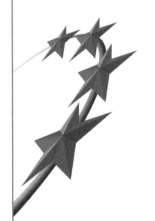

Covenant Healthcare

Milwaukee, Wis.

and total parenteral nutrition. Verbal orders for such drugs are no longer accepted by pharmacy or nursing.

Nursing Orientation. The orientation of new nurses to the medication use process was improved by addressing topics such as the order entry process, drug preparation and dispensing, availability of drug information, and medication safety initiatives.

Standardization of Insulin Sliding Scale Orders. The variability of sliding scale insulin orders has long been recognized as a source of dosing errors. Standardization provided consistency and a reduction in dosing confusion.

Physician Education. Safer prescribing habits, handwriting issues, and prescribing errors were addressed with physicians and other staff, individually and in groups. Specific error data were presented to identify dangerous abbreviations and unacceptable methods of expressing doses (i.e. trailing zeros for whole numbers or lack of using a leading zero for doses less than one).

Administration Set Labeling. A policy was developed that required the labeling of the distal ends of all administration sets so they are clearly visible on patients who are receiving multiple solutions via various routes of administration.

After implementating the Medication Error Reduction Program throughout Covenant, the Medication Safety Self-Assessment showed strong overall improvement in scores. The MERC and site-specific MSTs continue their work today, supported and recognized by the leaders of Covenant Healthcare.

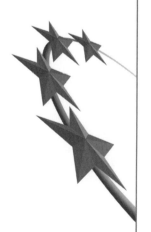

Covenant Healthcare
Milwaukee, Wis.

Computerized physician order entry has been proposed as one important method to reduce medication errors. Loyola University Medical Center used its existing "non-intelligent" commercial clinical information system installed in 1986 to facilitate system-wide computerized physician order entry for medications dispensed throughout the 540-bed hospital. Results demonstrated a dramatic decline in transcription errors and a positive impact on prescribing-related errors, as well as a significant reduction in unnecessary work. Further, it demonstrated that improvements in medication safety could be accomplished without investing in an expensive, new clinical information system.

A decision was made by the board of Loyola University Health System to initiate a system-wide improvement project to implement computerized physician order entry (CPOE) for medications throughout Loyola University Medical Center (LUMC). The clinical information system in use was Eclipsys TDS7000. The system had the capability to handle "non-intelligent" (i.e., no real-time decision support) CPOE, and use of this feature had been discussed intermittently since the time the system was purchased. Although studies of locally developed, intelligent clinical information systems at technology-intensive academic centers demonstrated that CPOE could be accomplished, it was unclear whether use of CPOE within an older generation, "non-intelligent," commercial information system would produce the desired outcomes.

At the initiation of the project, the potential benefits of CPOE were identified by the Quality Committee of the Loyola University Health System board as:

- major reduction in medication errors leading to improved quality and safety of care

- savings in pharmacist time

- fewer calls to residents, nurses, and ward clerks to clarify orders

- improved costs of therapy with use of preferred medication lists

- reduced legal liability

- change in resident, nursing, and ward clerk workflow

The executive medical director was assigned the responsibility of managing the CPOE project. The project team, led by a surgeon and a pulmonologist, was assembled and included faculty, residents, administrators, nurses, pharmacists, ward clerks, and information technology personnel. The effort was supported by the Center for Clinical Effectiveness, a quality improvement unit with a staff of 10 FTEs whose mission is to lead improvements in the quality and value of health care services rendered throughout the hospital.

The literature is replete with case studies of failed CPOE implementations that often resulted from inadequate management of the enormous change

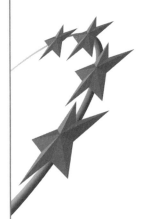

Loyola University Medical Center

Maywood, Ill.

involved in moving from paper-based ordering to computerization. With this awareness, we carefully planned our project activity and relied on the change management model of John Kotter from Harvard University, author of *"Leading Change"* and a renowned expert on change initiatives. A sense of urgency among board, senior management, and key physician leaders existed following discussion of the Institute of Medicine's findings and our review of internal data about medication errors. LUMC's institutional culture, existing structures necessary to proactively engage continuous quality improvement, and leadership support in steering the change effort helped to ensure the success of our initiative.

The project team extensively reviewed CPOE literature and had numerous conversations with leaders of two LUMC units that previously implemented CPOE on their own initiatives. Comprehensive, multidimensional education and marketing campaigns were undertaken with particular emphasis on reaching the clinical faculty, residents, and nurses because these stakeholders would be most affected by CPOE. Physician resistance was dramatically reduced once they reviewed actual, serious medication errors at LUMC and understood the potential benefits of this new process.

Pilot units were identified and physician and nursing leaders were actively engaged. The workflow of nurses and ward clerks was studied in detail and redesigned in an attempt to reduce the probability of failure at each step. The project team maintained extensive, ongoing discussions with residents, nurses, and clerks to acknowledge concerns and to identify ways to ease implementation. Some of the responses to end-user concerns included:

- customization of order entry screens and medication lists for individual departments
- availability of sufficient computers and printers on clinical units
- intervention of backup processes that could be used when the computer system was not operative
- processes for telephone, verbal, and STAT orders
- agreement that clerks and nurses would play a role helping physicians to learn the order entry process.

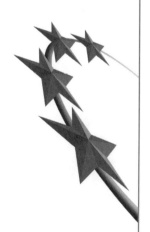

***Loyola
University
Medical Center***

Maywood, Ill.

CPOE was implemented progressively, beginning in intensive care units, then in all medical-surgical units. Regular, frequent project team meetings were held to make changes based on ongoing experience (i.e., numerous improvement cycles were employed). Regular reports were provided to senior administrators, physicians and nursing. The primary outcomes measure was the number of transcription-related medication errors intercepted by pharmacists and judged by a pharmacist to be of moderate or major clinical importance.

During the year prior to CPOE, transcription-related errors occurred at a mean rate of 72 per month and decreased to 57 per month during the pilot unit implementation. During the 15 months following hospital-wide implementation of CPOE, the error rate decreased 95% to 3.7 per month. Surprisingly, prescription-related errors decreased 36% from 151 to 96 per month. Although not explicitly studied, pharmacy staff noted a dramatic reduction in the time spent intervening on problematic medication orders.

This project demonstrated that transcription-related medication errors can be dramatically reduced through use of non-intelligent CPOE within an older clinical information system. Such a system, in fact, may have a positive impact on prescribing-related medication errors. In addition, CPOE has had a positive impact on the workload of the pharmacy staff. Other major benefits included the education of resident physicians, nurses, and ward clerks about patient safety as well as the benefits of participation in a multi-disciplinary quality improvement team.

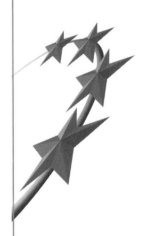

*Loyola
University
Medical Center*
Maywood, Ill.

Current standards of pain management present unique challenges to those working with inpatient psychiatric populations. Frequently, a merging of emotional and physical pain complicates pain management efforts. Recognizing this, the staff of Ohio State University & Harding Behavioral Healthcare and Medicine sought to increase their understanding and ability to manage the pain of psychiatric patients. They found that by initiating reassessment of pain within one-hour of the intervention, patient satisfaction with pain management improved by 23 percentage points.

This initiative was developed by Ohio State University (OSU) and Harding Behavioral Healthcare and Medicine (HBHM) to meet hospital and regulatory standards in the management of pain and to improve patient satisfaction with pain management. Focus groups were held with direct care providers to reevaluate the current approaches to pain management and to identify ways pain could be more effectively managed. The consensus of this group was that the practice of proactively inquiring about the effectiveness of a pain management intervention within one hour of its administration could impact patient perception and experience of pain. The staff also developed a systematized grouping of interventions such as relaxation techniques, deep breathing exercises, quiet areas, and warm baths or showers to supplement relief offered by medication.

Baseline data evaluation using regression analysis documented a 0.83 (95%CI) correlation between pain reassessment and satisfaction with pain management. Staff reassessment of pain within one-hour of intervention resulted in a 23 percentage point upward trend in satisfaction with pain management. Pain management has been added as an indicator on the balanced scorecard used to report outcomes. Ongoing efforts to measure the outcomes include, but are not limited to, the reduction of pain medication administration and the increased use of alternative methods to address pain issues.

The scope of the psychiatric pain management project was initially limited to inpatient psychiatric units. Since completion of this process, OSU & HBHM is embarking on a collaborative effort with the Ohio State University Medical Center Pain Management Program to address the psychologic component of pain within the general medical population.

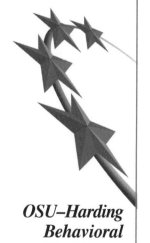

OSU–Harding
Behavioral
Healthcare
and Medicine

Columbus, Ohio

Ineffective treatment of pain has been extensively documented in health care literature as a common problem affecting nearly one-third to one-half of all patients. Despite the existence of best-practice evidence and comprehensive JCAHO pain management standards, it has been challenging to change pain management practices. PinnacleHealth System's Pain Management Committee was formed to ensure that all patients cared for by members of the system received quality pain management. The multifaceted plan implemented by the committee improved pain assessment, treatment, and documentation practices.

The Pain Management Committee was formed to ensure that PinnacleHealth System provided high quality care to patients experiencing pain. A multidisciplinary team representing all areas of the system was created to address this need. The committee met monthly to review pain-related issues and develop appropriate actions.

The first action taken by the committee was an extensive assessment of pain management at our system. This assessment allowed the committee to identify potential barriers to effective pain management and opportunities to improve both the assessment and interventions related to pain management. Recognizing that no single method or department could achieve a significant impact on system-wide issues, a multifaceted plan was developed. Initial efforts focused on: 1) increasing staff and physician knowledge about pain management, 2) improving pain assessment skills of staff and documentation practices, 3) reducing the use of meperidine for pain management, and 4) providing other pain management resources.

The committee formulated a policy and procedure for pain management to include in the administrative policy manual that clearly defines the system's commitment to pain relief as an integral part of comprehensive care requiring individualized treatment for total pain (physical, psychological, social, and spiritual). Another important step was the development of pain management practice guidelines for treatment of moderate to severe pain that includes: 1) standardized pain scales for adult, pediatric, neonatal, non-verbal, and non-English speaking patients, 2) information on pain assessment and types of pain, 3) pharmacologic and non-pharmacologic management of pain, and 4) information on opioid administration.

The committee identified that continued use of meperidine for pain management was not consistent with best practice evidence. As a result, meperidine guidelines were developed. Nursing representatives on the committee worked to revise automated documentation assessment screens, forms, and policies to improve documentation of pain management. A flow sheet for documenting complex pain management was developed for the critical care areas. The neonatal intensive care unit implemented the CRIES scale to assess postoperative pain in infants.

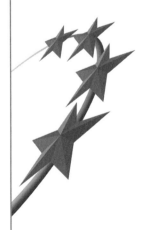

PinnacleHealth
Harrisburg, Pa.

These accomplishments were the cornerstone for educational activities throughout the year that included: 1) creation of a pain management display for Medical Education Day that was then rotated around the system hospitals and outpatient sites, 2) development of a self study pain management book for non-nursing staff, 3) creation of a pain management Intranet site, 4) development of patient education materials distributed to patients, and 5) participation in community events. A patient education pamphlet on pain management is given to all admitted patients.

Monthly documentation audits are performed and reported. Documentation of pain level and site on admission, using the standardized assessment scale, rose from 56% to 100% over a seven-month period. During that same period, documentation of postoperative assessment improved from 75% to 100%, and documentation of the use of non-pharmacologic interventions for pain management increased from 29% to 52%. Patient-controlled analgesia using meperidine decreased by 75% while use of other forms of injectable meperidine decreased by 88%.

Patient satisfaction scores have shown improvement. This indicator is difficult to analyze because of a change in the patient satisfaction survey process and tool that occurred around the time the project was implemented. Comparisons of scores on the two different surveys, however, indicate that the percentage of patients who were dissatisfied with their pain control dropped from 14% to 10%.

The committee continues to meet quarterly to discuss new issues and monitor the progress of the plan via the outcomes indicators. New areas have been identified for focusing future committee activities such as meeting the needs of special populations like patients in sickle cell crisis and with pancreatitis. Adverse medication reaction involving opioids is another area of interest that has generated additional attention.

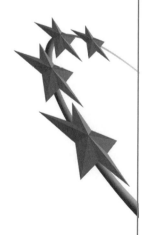

PinnacleHealth

Harrisburg, Pa.

One way hospitals have found to improve pain management is to place greater emphasis on education of medical and nursing staffs. The effectiveness of education can be measured by what one learns. It also can be evaluated in terms of how much of the acquired knowledge is retained over time. OSF Saint James – John W. Albrecht Medical Center developed a multidimensional approach to pain management education, including a class called "PAIN SMARTS!" To pass the course, participants were required to score more than 90% on a test administered at the end of the session. Ninety-seven percent of the nurses taking the test a year later scored 90% or better, indicating an impressive level of knowledge retention.

One recurring need that continued to surface as members of the Pain Team at OSF Saint James – John W. Albrecht Medical Center (OSF Saint James) discussed pain management was education. To determine what our nursing staff understood about pain management, we administered a shelf copy of a test from the Pain Clinical Manual (McAffery and Passero, 1999). The results demonstrated an average test score of less than 70%. With the goal of improving knowledge among registered and licensed practical nurses, a mandatory eight-hour educational seminar called, PAIN SMARTS! was developed.

The PAIN SMARTS! curriculum was design to include didactic learning and skill-development sessions in the areas that nurses lacked sufficient proficiency. Participants of the Pain Team divided some 15 pain topics into modules and served as faculty. Staff nurses attended sessions in groups of no more than 20 participants to maximize individualized learning. Skills stations covered areas of pain assessment, patient-controlled anesthesia, and epidural use. To successfully complete the course, nurses were required to demonstrate skill station competency and to pass the shelf test of the pain examination. A score of 90% was considered a passing grade.

Recognizing that traditional areas of pain management such as pathophysiology and pharmacology typically instill boredom in a classroom setting, we dveloped a Power Point® presentation and included visual and auditory cues to stimulate interest. This program subsequently won a Pinnacle Award from the Illinois Society for Healthcare Marketing and Public Relations for its creativity and innovative design.

The didactic sessions were punctuated with "problem-solvers," which were relevant and realistic examples of challenging pain situations. The nurses had to quickly synthesize the information they had learned while recommending solutions. The problem-solvers created a means by which to test multiple principles in pain management at the same time and provided immediate feedback on nursing comprehension.

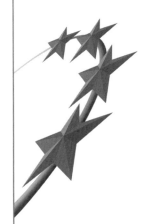

OSF Saint James–
John W. Albrecht
Medical Center

Pontiac, Ill.

In addition to raising awareness and knowledge, PAIN SMARTS! delivered several unanticipated benefits. Ownership was created because this was a program developed for and by OSF Saint James staff. We discovered another benefit as staff nurses taught the program and demonstrated the strength of their communication and leadership skills. After the training, the nursing faculty continued to serve as resources when difficult pain management problems were identified on a day-to-day basis.

Following the procedural changes and the educational sessions, OSF Saint James received the highest scores in pain assessment and documentation when measured among the six hospitals in the OSF system. More importantly, staff nurses attending PAIN SMARTS! helped the Pain Team identify numerous deficiencies and barriers that were previously unidentified. This further improved the quality of pain management.

The program has been an overwhelming success and is continued on a bi-annual basis for all new employees and incoming physicians. To assess the efficacy of the program, an exam was administered to all nursing staff one year after taking PAIN SMARTS! The results showed that 97% of nurses scored 90% or higher, demonstrating a remarkable degree of knowledge retention. The average nursing score is several points higher than the combined physician average!

The Pain Team has taken the philosophy that "people who are sitting on their laurels are wearing them on the wrong end." We continue to develop innovative approaches in education and pain management. Preliminary talks are underway to plan a new educational session called, PAIN SMARTS! – WE'RE BACK!

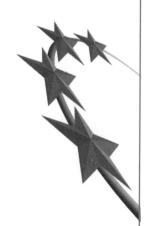

OSF Saint James–
John W. Albrecht
Medical Center

Pontiac, Ill.

A surgical delivery can be life-saving for mother and child if the baby is in distress, too large, or positioned the wrong way. But a C-section is major abdominal surgery. It is in the best interest of the patient to avoid C-sections, whenever possible. Based on JCAHO's ORYX and New York State's perinatal data, Rome Memorial Hospital's C-section rate was higher than the regional average. With the support of the hospital's quality council and board of trustees, a team of physicians, midwives, and nurses successfully reduced the C-section rate, cut length of stay by 8%, improved patient pain management and patient satisfaction, and reduced overall costs.

Rome Memorial Hospital is one of 20 hospitals across 15 counties that participate in the Central New York Perinatal Program, dedicated to improving the outcomes of pregnancy in Central New York. To reduce C-section rates, we first had to build awareness for the need. Statistics and graphs were reviewed quarterly at OB/GYN committee, quality council, and board of trustees meetings. Each physician also received individualized rates for the purpose of benchmarking against regional averages.

A C-section pathway, associated nursing care plans, and teaching documents, were developed. The most current standards of care and educational articles were consistently distributed to physicians and midwives.

In the true spirit of collaboration, the project engaged physicians, midwives, nursing and expectant mothers, and partners. They identified that reducing the path to C-section rate reduction begins at the physician offices when prenatal care visits are scheduled. Physicians and midwives focused on patient education to encourage a trial of labor. They also discussed techniques that could be used to facilitate the labor process.

Using the findings of a regional hospital comparison survey and site visit, nursing staff developed a proactive approach to labor coaching that empowers the expectant mother and her partner to feel more in control. A certified Lamaze instructor taught staff and patients various techniques to encourage women through the challenges of labor. These approaches included: 1) developing and distributing educational tools, 2) using birthing balls and stools to position women for birth, 3) involving physical therapists and water-birth specialists, 4) instructing women on ambulation and movement while in labor, and 5) using relaxation techniques.

The nursing staff was enthusiastic about the project. It gave them tools to provide assistance to the patients in their care. The initial investment of the program was $800 for an education video, birthing stool, and three birthing balls. The staff volunteered their time to learn the techniques because they believed that the project would benefit their patients.

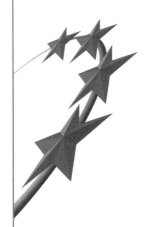

Rome Memorial Hospital

Rome, N.Y.

The performance improvement project generated the desired outcome of significantly reducing Rome Memorial Hospital's C-section rates. Surveys found that the proactive approaches not only reduced our rates, but also helped improve pain management in laboring mothers. Patients reported lower pain levels on the pain scale. With fewer mothers requiring the typical four-day stay after a C-section, the maternity department's average length of stay decreased 8%.

All of the stakeholders benefited from the project. The hospital reduced its costs. The nurses are more satisfied with their job performance because they can be more proactive in coaching women through labor. The physicians and midwives have patients who are more satisfied. Patients who have a natural birth are better able to take care of themselves and their newborn after delivery. They are at lower risk of post-delivery infection and pain. Through continuing education, use of labor coaching techniques, and focused awareness, the nurses, physicians, and midwives expect long term success in maintaining our C-section rates.

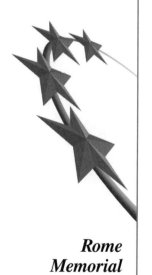

Rome
Memorial
Hospital
Rome, N.Y.

The prevalence of heart failure in the United States has increased steadily over the past 30 years and now affects nearly 5 million adults. Approximately 500,000 new cases are identified each year. While heart failure is treatable, one in five people with heart failure die within one year, mostly because of the failure to diagnose. In an effort to improve both patient and financial outcomes, a collaborative effort was made within the PinnacleHealth System to develop and implement a comprehensive Outpatient Heart Failure Program. A multidisciplinary team developed a standardized method for evaluating, treating, and monitoring patients. As a result, the 30-day readmission rate was cut from 22% to 8%, the 90-day readmission rate declined from 38% to 14%, and annual costs were reduced $500,000 for the first year.

Heart failure was the number one admitting diagnosis for persons over the age of 65 when PinnacleHealth System initiated the Outpatient Heart Failure Program. Class III and IV heart failure patients were hospitalized an average of five times a year with an average cost of $9,607 per patient per admission. Patient perception of quality of life (QOL) was affected by repeat hospitalizations and the ordeal of handling their new medical regimen. Length of stay (LOS) was 8.0 days. The rate of readmission within 30 days was 22%, and the 90 days readmission rate was 38%.

A multidisciplinary team included physician members from internal medicine, family practice, and cardiology; staff from case management, utilization review, and social services; and representatives from cardiovascular, patient care, financial services, home care, and dietary. The team developed the following goals: 1) reduce heart failure readmissions to acute care; 2) reduce length of stay; 3) increase appropriate use of ACE inhibitors, warfarin and/or beta blockers; 4) increase patient perception of quality of life; 5) improve inpatient education about diet/weight/medications; 6) improve documentation; and 7) reduce cost per case of management heart failure patients.

The team developed a four-tiered program that includes heart failure home care, in-home telemanagement, heart failure clinics, and cardiac rehabilitation. Criteria for enrollment were developed for each program. Patients are seen by the heart failure case manager who evaluates functional capacity using the New York Heart Association Functional Classification system, identifies co-morbidities including prior heart failure admission, and ensures completion of the QOL survey. A disease management assessment is completed. In-hospital management including appropriate use of ACE inhibitor, beta blocker, and warfarin is reviewed. The patient is also evaluated by the social worker to identify any psychosocial issues.

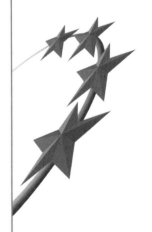

PinnacleHealth
Harrisburg, Pa.

Based on this information, the patient is enrolled in the appropriate management program. The patient receives extensive education to promote self-management starting in the hospital and continuing after discharge. The case manager coordinates education with nursing staff, dietary, and social services. This education includes lessons on administering medications, diet, symptoms of heart failure, heart failure disease process, and interaction with primary care providers. Consistent education materials across the continuum of services were developed to reduce patient confusion.

Through the efforts of this team and because of the support extended to its mission, we were able to increase patient perception of QOL, as measured by the Illness Effects Questionnaire. The average initial score of 78 indicated significant distress. After 12 weeks on the program, the average score was 42 (minimal distress). In addition, we reduced the 30 day readmission rate from 22% to 8% and the 90 day readmission rate from 38% to 14%. Length of stay decreased from 8.0 days to 6.5 days, and the average cost per heart failure admission decreased from $9,607 to $6,166. We achieved an initial year cost reduction of over $500,000, and cost reductions of over $100,000 in subsequent years.

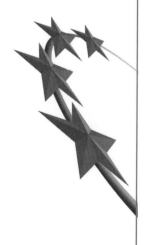

After negative publicity about infection control in hospitals, the JCAHO and other regulatory agencies are reviewing practices more closely. Finding no recognized threshold for a "good" antibiotic resistant organism rate in long term acute care hospitals against which to compare their outcomes, Spartanburg Hospital for Restorative Care asked, "Can we perform better?" With support from senior leadership, a multidisciplinary team used basic infection control principles to reduce the facility's nosocomial antibiotic resistant organism rates by as much as 56%.

Senior leaders at Spartenburg Hospital for Restorative Care (SHRC) were eager to know that were we doing all we could to minimize the threat of antibiotic-resistant organisms (AROs). Antibiotic resistant infections like methicillin/oxicillan-resistant staphylococcus aureus (MRSA/ORSA) and vancomycin-resistant enterococcus (VRE) became hot-topics when television icon Rosie O'Donnell contracted MRSA after a minor procedure and raised awareness of this problem. In light of the media frenzy, we immediately turned our attention to infection-control practices.

The Performance Management Council commissioned an interdisciplinary performance improvement team to assess the hospital's infection control practices and its effect on nosocomial ARO rates. After weeks of intense research on the subject, the team kept coming back to the same conclusion: If you want to minimize the spread of AROs, you have to identify patients who carry the organisms and then isolate them from the rest of the patient population. This simple principle was not new or cutting-edge. "Identify, then isolate" is an infection-control practice nearly as old as the profession.

Armed with the team's findings and her own tenacity, the infection control practitioner took a proposal to SHRC's administration, medical executive committee, and board of directors. She asked hospital leadership to approve a new infection control program that entailed proactively screening all patients on admission for AROs and then isolating those patients who tested positive. Infection control received approval to carry out the program for 12 months and then evaluate its effectiveness.

The team rolled out massive education on the proactive ARO screening program during which they also reinforced knowledge of standard and isolation precautions. Those patients that tested positive for ARO are placed in isolation per SHRC's infection control guidelines. Education is then provided to the patients and their significant others regarding the ARO and isolation precautions. Early identification and isolation of patients carrying an ARO significantly reduces the risk of transmission.

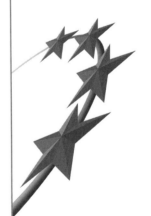

Spartanburg Hospital for Restorative Care

Spartanburg, S.C.

Success was almost instantaneous. In the first month of screening, nosocomial MRSA/ORSA and VRE rates dropped dramatically. At the end of 12 months, this initiative reduced the nosocomial MRSA/ORSA rate by 55.9% and the nosocomial VRE rate by 48.4%.

Implementing a hospital-wide screening of this nature is both time and cost intensive. The total cost, including labor and supplies for the first full year of screening was estimated at $136,223.

Based on our substantial decrease in nosocomial ARO rates, SHRC estimates that it prevented 16 patients from infection with MRSA/ORSA and five patients from infection with VRE. A special report published by the Society for Healthcare Epidemiology of America, suggests that the average attributable cost for one incident of MRSA/ORSA is $35,367. The same report estimates costs for an incident of VRE at $27,000. Based on these statistics, SHRC prevented approximately $700,872 in ARO related costs representing a net savings of $564,649.

This project proved one of the simplest yet significant performance improvement initiatives undertaken by SHRC in its eight-year history. Though the proactive screening program entails significant time and resources, the infection control department is able to justify the cost with overwhelming benefit. Senior leadership within the organization resolved to continue financial and administrative support for the proactive ARO screening program. This commitment ensures that SHRC will continue to protect patients against the threat of antibiotic-resistant organisms.

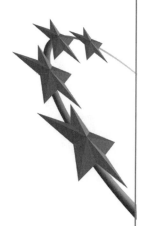

Spartanburg Hospital for Restorative Care
Spartanburg, S.C.

The treatment patients need for pulmonary conditions is administered through metered-dose inhalers that deliver the prescribed dosages from a canister that holds the medication. If the course of treatment is discontinued before the canister's content is used, the medication is wasted. This led a team at St. Joseph's Hospital to develop a protocol that allows respiratory therapists and registered nurses to administer treatments from a common canister, using disposable mouthpieces for each patient. This common canister protocol, along with education, resulted in enhanced outcomes and an estimated $30,000 in savings the first year.

At St. Joseph's Hospital, respiratory therapists and registered nurses administer treatments to patients with pulmonary diseases and respiratory problems. We recognized the need to improve both staff and patient education about the proper administration of treatment with metered-dose inhalers (MDI). We also saw an opportunity to reduce waste by providing spacers with a one-way valve that would allow us to use a common canister without the attendant concerns about contamination or spread of infection to patients.

Two units participated in the three-month trial using the new procedures. First, we charted the current process and determined areas of breakdown that resulted in suboptimal therapy or staff confusion. We then educated the staff. Respiratory therapists always provided the first MDI treatment for a patient and demonstrated correct procedures to RNs so they could observe and learn how to educate patients to self-administer the MDI. A MDI patient education form was developed as a tool so patients received consistent instruction.

Staff from pharmacy and respiratory therapy worked to develop the protocol for using the common canister. We also developed a plan for ordering a supply of our commonly used MDIs every week, which were to be stored in a special box kept in a common location on each nursing unit. Fewer inhalers were lost as a result. After receiving the patient education tool, patients were more confident about correct administration techniques. There were no documented patient infections resulting from use of the common canisters with spacers. To date, the common canister protocol is used hospital-wide and we have projected the cost savings to be $30,000 annually.

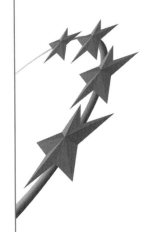

St. Joseph's Hospital

Elmira, N.Y.

Falling is the fifth leading cause of death and the second leading cause of accidental death among people over age 65. Sharp Grossmont Hospital's progressive care unit recognized that by identifying at-risk patients and making all staff more conscious of how falls occur, fall incidents could be reduced. The program focused on educating people about commonly overlooked factors that contribute to fall accidents. During the first year of the program, the number of falls in the unit dropped to 40 from 65.

Patient safety and prevention of falls are integral parts of providing the highest quality nursing care. Because of a significant increase in patient falls in the progressive care unit (PCU), Sharp Grossmont Hospital staff revamped its existing policy to ensure patient safety.

We analyzed contributing factors and identified precautionary measures that would prevent falls from occurring in the future. We then established new practices that would help us remain alert to patients who were at risk for falls. All patients at risk for falls are identified using the Schmidt Fall Risk Assessment Tool. We update staff during shift reports to inform all caregivers of those patients who are identified as being at risk. Teamwork is instrumental in the success of the Fall Prevention Program. We all work together: staff, patients, their families and other departments such as physical therapy, transporters, and discharge planners. The program improved the continuous communications needed to ensure patient safety. We found that patients and family members needed more information about measures that could be taken to reduce the likelihood of falls. We identified the need to train staff to be more fall-conscious and to publicize risk factors and increase staff awareness.

Since implementing the Fall Prevention Program, the number of falls in the PCU dropped from 65 to 40 in a year. Equally impressive, there were no incidents of repeat falls by patients in the entire year following the initiation of the program. The staff has become fall-conscious and use of the tools has become routine. Other hospital units soon adopted the program, and it is now being instituted hospital-wide. It also is included in the education classes of the new nursing grad program with the goal of increasing awareness of the risk of patient falls among new nurses during their orientation process.

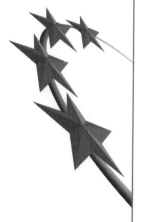

Sharp Grossmont Hospital

La Mesa, Calif.

The use of visual cues to warn staff of safety risks is not uncommon but Carondelet St. Joseph's Hospital invented a novel approach for identifying patients at risk for falling. Ruby slippers are placed on the feet of these patients. Reminiscent of the slippers that were worn by Dorothy in the Wizard of Oz, the slippers remind staff that they can make a difference in patient safety. Even before employees were trained in fall prevention, incidence of patient falls decreased due to the "buzz" the ruby slippers created.

The Ruby Slippers Program was prompted by a noted increase in the number of falls on the med/surg and rehab units of Carondelet St. Joseph's Hospital. We decided to take a very proactive approach to patient safety and implement a risk reduction program that would involve all associates and all disciplines in preventing patient falls.

The first indication of our potential for success was revealed once we began discussing the proposed project on our units. The suggestion that ruby slippers would help to reduce falls attracted attention. Within months, fewer patients were falling simply because of the heightened awareness of staff.

We found the perfect red slippers with the help of central supply, and once they were placed on patients' feet; incidents of falls dropped, patients did not.

Our discussions were not limited to employees on these units. We began alerting physicians to our program and spreading the word about patient safety throughout St. Joseph's and St. Mary's, another hospital in our system. We made a Power Point® teaching program available on our Intranet so all staff could learn about fall prevention and patient safety.

The ruby slippers remind patients that we care about their safety. The strength of the visual cue reminds staff that we are all responsible for patient safety.

Ruby Slippers is being adapted and piloted for use in the St. Joseph's Hospital Emergency Department. ED patients at high risk are those who are likely to elope before being thoroughly assessed for risk to self or others. These patients will be given red exam gowns, instead of red slippers, to wear. The name of this program is "Ruby R*ED."

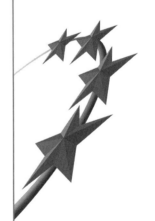

*Carondelet
St. Joseph's
Hospital*

Tucson, Ariz.

The Surgical Learning Institute, located at Florida Hospital Celebration Health, is a premier center for hands-on surgical instruction. The prime objective of the institute is to develop and disseminate surgical knowledge and techniques to the global community through state-of-the-art teleconferencing technology. This visionary project was jointly conceptualized by industrial innovators and surgeons, and has become a new standard in telemedical surgical education.

Florida Hospital Celebration Health serves as a living laboratory for health care change and is an international show site for telesurgery and telementoring. The setting of the Surgical Learning Institute is one in which participants gain hands-on knowledge and understanding of specific surgical techniques as well as how to properly use new equipment and technology.

The setting allows for experimentation, research, and education related to 21st century surgical skills improvement. Each learning station mirrors a typical endoscopically-equipped operating suite and is outfitted with the latest teleconferencing technology. This integration allows connectivity with any external environment, and it is the ideal distance learning model. The interactive surgical learning experience can be shared dynamically in a teleconference forum or can be captured on a variety of digital media to be shared worldwide with other surgeons. An open forum assures dynamic content-sharing to the global surgical community.

Surgeons, educators, and industry partners significantly expand their knowledge and practice bases in multiple surgical disciplines through educational workshops, conferences and symposia. Participants of surgical educational courses master minimally invasive operative techniques on cadaveric models. The education and skills acquired by participants in this learning environment positively impact thousands of patients through improved surgical outcomes.

The Surgical Learning Institute provides a technology-rich environment for surgeons and health care innovators to develop new technologies and procedures that benefit the surgical community. We integrate multiple teaching models into a single experience that is dynamic. The success of this project has been measured by our ability to disseminate the latest surgical knowledge and skill to the global surgical community utilizing a distance learning model.

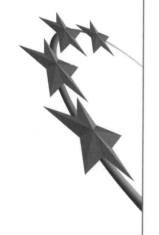

Florida Hospital Celebration Health

Celebration, Fla.

The Road to Safe Surgery was developed by Carondelet St. Joseph's Hospital to facilitate compliance with documentation of core perioperative processes. All processes must be complete before the patient enters the surgical suite. After implementing the program, the compliance rate for documentation rose to 100%. The project was so successful, a surgeon borrowed the concepts to implement at a competing hospital.

A multidisciplinary team was formed to review the flow process of perioperative patients at Carondelet St. Joseph's Hospital. Our emphasis was on core components necessary to meet compliance with JCAHO standards of care. Benchmark data was identified by the team and provided to the perioperative unit director. The team identified three opportunities for immediate improvement: 1) signed informed consent by the patient, surgeon, and anesthesiologist, 2) a history and physical exam completed within seven days of surgery, and 3) surgical site verification.

The recommendation was to develop a system that would insure 100% compliance with the three identified core processes. A systematic action plan was initiated by the unit director and the clinical nurse educator to improve performance and compliance. The plan came to be known as "The Road to Safe Surgery."

At the outset, it was understood that for the program to succeed, all stakeholder groups needed to be consulted. The following groups were involved in offering input into the program: 1) medical staff including primary care physicians, surgeons, and anesthesiologists; 2) perioperative staff; 3) hospital administration; and 4) surgical patients. As a result of the collaborative process, several changes took place. The informed surgical consent form was modified to include a section for the anesthesiologist to obtain the patient consent for anesthesia. Policy and procedures for consent, history and physical exam requirements, and site/side marking were reviewed, updated and implemented. In addition, senior leadership established the consequences for noncompliance with core processes. Guidelines for disciplinary action were set up in advance of program implementation. A lime green tracking form was developed to monitor compliance.

The next step in the planning process was to provide education for senior leadership, patients, perioperative and medical staffs regarding the requirements. A patient brochure was distributed to every surgical patient during pre-admission testing.

A storyboard was put together and set up in a strategic place for all stakeholders to see. The patient brochure, program requirements to meet compliance, and the start date also were displayed on the storyboard. Presentations were made to medical executive board members, senior

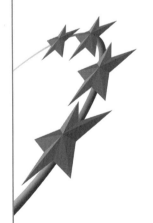

*Carondelet
St. Joseph's
Hospital*

Tucson, Ariz.

administrators, and perioperative and medical staffs. A self-learning packet was prepared to provide more details and information on the rationale behind the requirements. Policies and guidelines were attached to the packet so everyone could became familiar with them before the program was implemented.

The final phase before implementation of the plan was to provide some visual cues so that the staff could tell from a glance whether the chart was complete. This was done by mounting large clips to every stretcher to hold either a red or green 3" x 6" laminated tag. A red tag (STOP) indicates an incomplete chart whereas a green tag (GO) signals a complete chart. A green tag must be displayed on the bed before the patient can proceed to the surgical suite.

When the procedures were launched, two traffic lights were installed as reminders to the staff that the program was officially implemented. Now the patients arrive at the holding with a red tag on their stretcher. As each of three reviews is completed, a check mark is placed on the lime green tracking form. Once all documentation is done and the form is complete, the red tag is changed to a green tag. The tracking form is saved and used for data collection.

Before implementation of the program, the compliance rate for chart completion was 79%. Because we did not have a satisfactory process for dealing with noncompliance, it was challenging to deal with the issue of incomplete charts. By instituting the Road to Safe Surgery, there is no room for compromise with such requirements. We now enjoy 100% compliance and the cooperation of all parties concerned with patient safety. We vigorously monitor compliance.

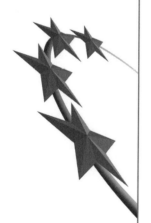

*Carondelet
St. Joseph's
Hospital*

Tucson, Ariz.

Transfusion-free medicine uses state-of–the-art techniques to minimize blood loss before, during, and after treatments for many illnesses. This sophisticated approach permits doctors to care for patients without using additional blood products because each patient retains enough of his or her own blood for medical procedures. Columbia Memorial Hospital implemented the Transfusion-Free Medicine and Surgery Program to reduce or eliminate the inherent risks associated with the transfusion of blood and to offer an alternative to individuals who, for religious or personal reasons, refuse the transfusion of blood or blood products. As a result, blood transfusions have decreased from a monthly average of 128 units to 87 units.

The vision of a Transfusion-Free Medicine and Surgery Program began to form as a small committee of individuals began looking at the use of blood and blood products at Columbia Memorial Hospital. This committee was assembled after our director of transfusion services noted an increasing number of articles in professional journals that discussed the multiple risks associated with blood transfusion. In addition to risk of transmission of infectious diseases such as hepatitis and HIV, it was noted that blood transfusions depress the immune system. As a result, patients who receive a transfusion during surgery have a higher incidence of postoperative infection, longer hospitalization, and for some types of cancer, a higher rate of recurrence.

It was initially the intention of the committee to investigate the use of blood by the surgery department and develop a program that would reduce the number of transfusions given by our surgeons. But it quickly became apparent that this program could benefit all patients, and it was noted to be of particular importance to Jehovah's Witnesses in our community whose religion prohibits receiving the transfusion of blood or blood products.

The program quickly became a two-fold project: 1) to provide alternatives to blood transfusion for all patients who have personal or religious objection, and 2) to eliminate the need for transfusions for all patients. This is performed by limiting the amount of blood a patient loses before, during, and after treatments.

A new larger multidisciplinary team was the formed. The team continued to gather data on bloodless medicine to include non-blood management techniques. Several specialists were brought into the facility to provide educational sessions for our medical staff. Our multidisciplinary team also made site visits to a hospital that had implemented a bloodless medicine program. Policies and procedures were reviewed, bloodless medical and surgical techniques were discussed, and the instrumentation used in non-blood management was demonstrated.

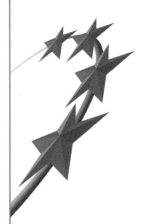

*Columbia
Memorial
Hospital*

Hudson, N.Y.

Our program coordinator attended educational sessions at the Bloodless Medicine and Surgery Institute in Cleveland, Ohio. Policies and procedures were developed. Our laboratory instituted micro sampling, a process involving the use of smaller blood collection tubes for diagnostic testing, and the anesthesiology department adopted a procedure called acute normovolemic hemodilution. This procedure involves withdrawing the patient's own blood after the induction of anesthesia, replacing the blood with a diluting fluid during surgery, and returning the patient's blood at the conclusion of the surgical procedure. Both procedures are designed to minimize the amount of blood a patient loses. Columbia Memorial Hospital purchased its first "cell saver," which allows surgeons to collect blood being shed during a surgical case, cleanse, and return the blood to the patient.

To ensure that these procedures met the tenets of religious beliefs, a group of elders from the Jehovah's Witness church was invited to review and provide feedback on our program. Our program coordinator then conducted staff education. This training included education on the philosophy of bloodless medicine, standards of care, techniques to minimize blood loss; the beliefs of Jehovah's Witnesses; and our newly developed policies and procedures.

In preparation for using the new cell saver technology, post-anesthesia care unit (PACU) nurses received training on the set-up, operation, trouble shooting, and breakdown of equipment. These nurses became resident experts and offered training to all surgical services nurses. To ensure competency in the operation of this equipment, PACU nurses also developed a biannual competency-testing program that each surgical services nurse is required to complete.

After over one year of planning, Columbia Memorial Hospital became one of only 100 hospitals in the United States and one of only seven hospitals in New York state to offer a comprehensive bloodless medicine and surgical program to its patients.

Blood transfusions have decreased. Monthly averages have fallen from an average of 128 units transfused to 87 units transfused. During one year, all patients having elective total joint replacements have been cared for without the transfusion of a single unit of blood. In past years it was customary practice for these patients to receive one to three units of blood in the post-operative period depending on the type of surgery preformed. Through education and the use of blood sparing medical and surgical techniques, we now offer this exceptional state-of-the-art care to all of our patients.

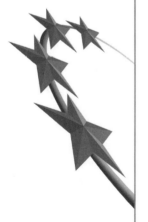

*Columbia
Memorial
Hospital*

Hudson, N.Y.

CHAPTER 6
PERFORMANCE IMPROVEMENT

PERFORMANCE IMPROVEMENT

Why do patients travel to destinations outside of the service area to receive health care services? This perplexing question was asked by Columbus Regional Hospital after it opened a Breast Health Center and discovered a significant number of women continued to go elsewhere for routine screenings. In this instance, Columbus Regional Hospital learned there were service-oriented deficiencies that needed to be remedied before it could hope to win the confidence of women in the community. After restructuring service delivery and adding a nurse navigator, growing demand for services offered by the Breast Health Center validated the wisdom of listening to customers.

A s part of our ongoing commitment to women's health and the community we serve in south central Indiana, Columbus Regional Hospital (CRH) created a Breast Health Center to provide screening mammograms for women. Yet, a large number of women continued to leave the area for routine and diagnostic treatments. We conducted a survey of 625 consumers in a seven county area and found that although 56.7% were aware that the hospital offered mammography services, only 25.3% perceived this service to be a strength of the hospital. We then conducted focus group research involving women who had received breast care services at institutions outside of the Columbus area. This inquiry revealed that perceptions relating to the convenience, responsiveness, and coordination of care at Columbus Regional Hospital's Breast Health Center influenced decisions to seek care elsewhere.

We assembled a multidisciplinary team comprised of two physician champions and representatives from the hospital mammography service, radiology department, and administration to develop an improvement plan. We used "Force Field Analysis" to analyze the forces that drive and restrain change. This helped us to anticipate what we would need to do to achieve the desired state of providing quality service, as defined by the customer, in one location and in a timely manner.

Our goal was to provide comprehensive breast health education, screening and diagnostic procedures, treatment alternatives, and referrals through the Breast Health Center to meet the needs of women in the community. Key quality characteristics that were identified as necessary to meet patient needs included: 1) speed and efficiency, 2) patient involvement in decisions, 3) access to information, 4) seamless delivery and a process that flows smoothly, 5) confidence that someone is overseeing the patient's care, 6) help in navigating the system, and 7) coordination so that everyone involved in the patient's care is informed and aware.

The overall intent of the improvement effort was to address these requirements, increase patient satisfaction, and improve the perceptions of our services.

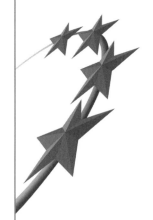

Columbus
Regional
Hospital

Columbus, Ind.

We addressed the following areas:

Relocate Screening and Diagnostic Services to One Location. The Breast Health Center was originally designed to do screening mammograms. Women needing additional diagnostic studies were referred to the hospital. Since relocating all of the screening and diagnostic services to one location, there is now greater perceived continuity of care for patients who require diagnostic services following screening mammograms. There is also a stronger feeling of cohesiveness among the team members.

Allow Self-Referrals For Screening Mammograms. Early detection is a key in the treatment of breast disease. We determined that we would accept self-referrals for screening mammograms, thereby removing one step in the process of accessing this important service. Physicians in our community resisted this proposal, and it was important to be sensitive and responsive to their concerns. We did not want our decision to cause them to stop referring their patients to our Breast Health Center. We learned that physicians were concerned that self-referred patients could fall through the cracks and not receive follow-up care. We came up with protocols to address this. Each woman who schedules a mammogram is asked if she has a family physician. If she does, we notify that physician's office. If the patient does not have an existing relationship with a doctor, the Breast Health Center assists in finding one.

Provide Timely, Team-oriented Service. The team agreed that a patient needing diagnostic services would want to have all testing completed as quickly as possible, with results returned rapidly. We responded by restructuring our delivery processes and staffing. Screening mammograms are offered in the mornings on Monday, Wednesday and Thursday and all day on Tuesday and Friday. Once a month, we offer Saturday morning appointments. One radiologist is assigned to mammography for the week to read films in the Breast Health Center. This is done to ensure that the patient can speak with the same physician if additional tests are required.

Patients needing additional imaging and/or biopsies to confirm suspicious findings from screening mammograms can have these scheduled right away because diagnostic imaging is scheduled three afternoons a week on Monday, Wednesday and Thursday.

Although centralized scheduling in the hospital was efficient, it did not allow for the flexibility that is sometimes necessary when a specific patient has needs that should be addressed immediately. The scheduler now assigned to the Breast Health Center can push the schedule to meet these needs.

Surgeons reworked their call schedules to be available to meet with radiologists or patients between noon and 1 p.m. on diagnostic days. This block of time

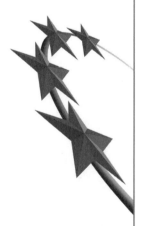

Columbus Regional Hospital

Columbus, Ind.

is held to guarantee that a surgeon is available to talk with the patient within 24 hours of diagnostic testing. Pathologists redistributed their workloads to accommodate needs of patients and physicians of the Breast Health Center. Now, when we need to schedule a biopsy late in the day, pathology responds with a willingness to accommodate patient needs. Pathology results are available the morning after most biopsies.

Create a Nurse Navigator Position. A nurse navigator is assigned the responsibility of assisting patients with coordination of their care, education, and access to cancer resources. If a patient needs to return for diagnostic testing after a routine mammogram, the nurse makes phone calls to the patient and referring physician.

The nurse navigator role proved to be effective and provides a single contact for the patient or physician to obtain information. The intent of this role has remained focused on helping the patient through the complex health care system at a vulnerable time in her life. The nurse navigator phones the patient the evening of, and the morning after, a diagnosis to provide reassurance and support. The nurse remains with the patient during all phases of diagnosis, including appointments with surgeons and oncologists. In addition, the nurse navigator meets the patient on the morning of her operation. Patients are encouraged to call the nurse navigator with questions. The nurse navigator has computer access to more than 1,200 articles that can be referenced and printed out for patients, and she can provide referrals to plastic surgeons, oncologists, other medical specialists, and outlets for products/services that may be needed during treatment such as wigs, prostheses, and skin care products.

We wanted to create a clinically integrated approach to breast health that included radiology, breast surgery, plastic surgery, oncology, and other medical specialties, but our focus has always been on the patient and her needs for convenience, comfort, support, and peace of mind. Our responsiveness has contributed positively to public perception about the Breast Health Center. As women relate their experiences to other women, "word-of-mouth" advertising supports our marketing efforts. Volumes have steadily risen. In the first year, 4,836 mammograms were performed; within five years, that number doubled. The growth has slowed, but it still continues in an upward direction and is on plan with our projections.

Although we have recently purchased new technology that enables us to improve the quality of our services, our team's human effort to respond quickly and communicate effectively has clearly been the main key to improving patient perception of the quality of our caring.

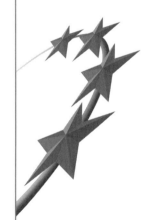

Columbus Regional Hospital

Columbus, Ind.

Northwestern Memorial Hospital's strategic goal of delivering the Best Patient Experience from the patient's perspective is deeply embedded in the culture of this organization. A pilot project to serve as a model to support the Best Patient Experience was initiated, and an entire floor of the outpatient pavilion that delivers diagnostic services to approximately 120,000 patients annually was selected as the site. Using patient feedback and the unique perspectives of team representatives, Northwestern Memorial Hospital improved patient access and flow, turnaround and availability of medical reports, and patient satisfaction with the overall experience of care.

The Best Patient Experience pilot project at Northwestern Memorial Hospital (NMH) was developed to advance our strategic goal of delivering the Best Patient Experience from the patient's perspective. The Best Patient Experience means that we provide what patients want, when they want it, how they want it, and where they want to receive it. It means delivering the best possible outcomes, treating each of our patients like family members, and ensuring 100% patient satisfaction. It means providing patient care services in a warm, welcoming and comforting environment. It means always exceeding patient expectations.

An entire floor of the hospital's outpatient pavilion was selected as the pilot site. It reports to one director and one vice president and is home to a variety of diagnostic departments including nuclear medicine, nuclear cardiology, stress testing, Holter monitoring, ECG services, echo lab, vascular lab, pulmonary function, cardiac catheterization lab, and electrophysiology lab.

A steering committee that included management staff from departments on the floor, patient representatives, a physician representative, and the director of professional services was challenged to "think outside the box" to develop the project plan. The team conducted face-to-face patient interviews to identify opportunities for satisfaction improvement and potential barriers to implementation. Patients told us the registration process was too much of a hassle; it was difficult to find the department; there was no communication regarding delays; and wait times between appointments and procedures were too long.

Patient experience was analyzed from point of entry through bill payment. It became clear the team should think less departmentally and more organizationally. When barriers to improvement were identified, ad hoc committee members were added until the barriers were removed. What began as a local project soon became hospital-wide, including representatives from quality, finance, facilities, environmental services, and patient transportation.

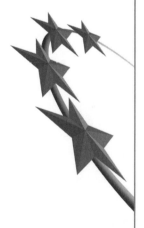

Northwestern Memorial Hospital

Chicago, Ill.

Three key areas for improvement emerged: patient flow, access and information flow. The steering committee divided the project into three phases.

Phase I. We simplified access amd navigation of the hospital campus by improving signage and revamping the patient check-in process. We went from six points of access on the 8th floor to two check-in points, both adjacent to our main visitor elevators. We separated the greeting and check-in functions from patient scheduling to provide visitors with an attentive and personalized arrival experience.

We outfitted front desk staff with the same uniforms as customer service officers stationed in the main lobbies of the hospital for a consistent and familiar image that would be recognized throughout the medical center as information resources. An innovation that continues to fascinate and please our patients is the electronic seating chart. When patients check in, we note their seating locations in the waiting area, and when the time to call a patient for his or her procedure arrives, our staff approaches the patient and greets him or her quietly by name. This eliminates the uncomfortable practice of shouting the names and compromising patient confidentiality. Staff members escort patients to procedure rooms.

Patient escorts were outfitted with intercom headsets. They know which patient is to be called next and are aware of delays a patient may encounter. After a procedure, patients are escorted back to the public area. A customer service coordinator communicates directly with patients who have waited more than 10 minutes from the time of a scheduled appointment. The customer service coordinator serves as liaison between the waiting area and the procedure areas and is empowered to solve problems, attend to any special needs, and coordinate special services.

Phase II. During this phase, we focused primarily on being able to provide non-emergent, routine outpatient appointments within one day and final interpretive reports within 24 hours. To accomplish this, we extended our hours of operation by offering evening and weekend appointments. We consolidated departmental scheduling, creating a central scheduling office for the 8th floor and cross-training personnel to schedule for any procedure offered.

Phase III. The final phase addressed being able to rapidly access diagnostic reports via the electronic medical record system. By doing this, we dramatically reduced calls coming into diagnostic departments requesting reports. At the same time, we streamlined the registration process so approximately 80% of registrations are handled at the time of scheduling. This eliminates the need for patients to be transferred to another department to complete their registration or make another call to register.

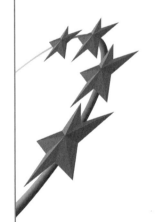

Northwestern Memorial Hospital

Chicago, Ill.

We established a Health Learning Center satellite in a public waiting area. There we provide educational materials, computers with Internet access and technical support for patient/visitor education, as well as information about NMH and the city of Chicago.

Historically, NMH has achieved high patient satisfaction scores. Within the first two quarters after implementing the Best Patient Experience pilot project, overall satisfaction rose 3.7 percentage points; reception desk scores rose 5.1 points; informed about delays scores rose 4.3 points; ease of check-in scores rose 3.1 points. Ninety percent of procedures are now scheduled within 1-2 days, down from the previous average of 7-10 days. Interpretive reports are now completed faster, with 80% of them done in 24 hours; previously fewer than 50% were completed in this time frame. Virtually 100% of reports are now available on our electronic medical record system, whereas none was available electronically prior to project implementation.

The Best Patient Experience pilot project created a greater spirit of teamwork between departments. Its success has been communicated to all in the organization and has resulted in an overwhelming sense of pride and an increased commitment to NMH's mission of Patients First. What is most meaningful is found in the comments received from patients themselves. As one recently wrote, "This was the best outpatient service I have ever received. I always feel like a guest here, not just a patient."

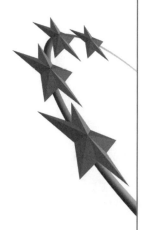

Northwestern Memorial Hospital

Chicago, Ill.

When patients, staff, and physicians of an emergency department are dissatisfied, it is challenging to know where and how to begin an improvement initiative. Sometimes it just makes sense to isolate a problem and plant the first step. That is how the director at Cape Canaveral Hospital responded when she pulled together a team to look at the triage and registration processes. Patients arriving to the emergency department were not the only ones who benefited when the average wait time (arrival to treatment) was reduced 85%. This accomplishment was a big boost to the morale of the entire department and initiated a series of improvements that caused satisfaction and spirits to soar.

A couple of years ago, the emergency department at Cape Canaveral Hospital ranked in the 12th percentile in patient satisfaction. Emergency department physicians and staff were dissatisfied. Morale was at an all-time low. Teamwork was basically nonexistent. It was clear that our department did not meet the vision statement of our organization, which says we are committed to "assuring quality care at competitive prices and the highest levels of patient satisfaction." The challenge was to decide where to begin. An analysis of the issues showed that patient volumes had increased dramatically while the processes used to provide treatment remained unchanged. This resulted in bottlenecks, overcrowding and long waits for treatment, and patient, staff and physician dissatisfaction.

A team composed of ED staff and physicians was convened to look at the triage and registration processes. Data showed the average wait time from sign-in to treatment was 90 minutes. The team streamlined the triage process and initiated bedside registration. Five months later results showed an 85% decrease in average wait times; the time from sign-in to treatment was 13.5 minutes, despite a 15% increase in volume. Patient complaints began to decrease and physician and staff morale started to improve.

This success generated enthusiasm and buy-in. Additional teams were assembled to address other performance improvement initiatives, including: 1) creation of an ED case manager position to facilitate patient discharge and follow-up, 2) implementation of an ED clinical information system, which included patient tracking, order entry, nurse documentation, and discharge instructions, 3) creation of a five-bed Express Care area to treat non-urgent patients faster, and 4) implementation of service culture training for the ED staff.

A Nursing Process Council moved to improve satisfaction and efficiency of the ED nursing staff by eliminating delays in the overall admission process. There has been a significant decrease in ED holding hours because of increased bed availability in all areas of the hospital.

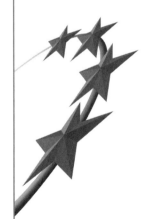

Cape Canaveral Hospital

Coco Beach, Fla.

One of the Emergency Nurses Standards of Care says, "Emergency nurses shall assure open and timely communication with emergency patients, their significant others and team members to ensure the occurrence of therapeutic interventions." We focused on the needs to keep patients informed, communicate delays, and include them in their treatment plan. Documentation parameters were built into the ED clinical information system to serve as reminders and facilitate data collection.

The impact of our improvement initiatives has been improved communication and cooperation internally and with staff in other departments. A culture that supports staff empowerment and collaboration has been established.

Amazing things began to happen as processes and bottlenecks improved. A strong sense of teamwork developed among everyone who works in the emergency department. Our staff satisfaction ranked at the 97th percentile within two years. Despite the current nursing shortage, we have no nurse vacancies and minimal turnover of staff.

Annual patient volumes have continued to soar and customer satisfaction has steadily improved. Within two years, patient satisfaction ranked at the 94th percentile and we handled a 23.8% increase in emergency department volume at the same time. The emergency department scored in the 97th percentile on the latest customer satisfaction survey. We are now a team of extraordinary people providing extraordinary care and service excellence at Cape Canaveral Hospital.

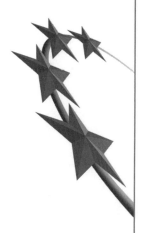

*Cape
Canaveral
Hospital*

Coco Beach, Fla.

With the increasing numbers of uninsured people seeking routine and emergent treatment from emergency departments, very few hospitals in America have escaped the trauma of ED overcrowding. Parma Community General Hospital took a unique approach to solve its overcrowding problem. A plan for active patient management was crafted after forming Healthcare Excellence through Action Teams (HEAT). By turning to HEAT, Parma dramatically improved patient satisfaction and reduced diversion hours.

W ill your ER be there for you? This question was posed in an article featured in Cleveland's *The Plain Dealer.* The newspaper's investigative series revealed that ambulance diversions have quadrupled throughout the country as a result overcrowded emergency departments (ED). "Hospitals have never held more promise for people who need life-saving treatments," it began. "But first, you have to get in the door."

At the time the article appeared, Parma Community General Hospital's ED, which sees about 42,000 patients a year, was struggling with many performance indicators. In order to remain true to our mission "to provide access to affordable, quality health care to everyone in need of our services," the ED doors must stay open. While making expansion plans to accommodate more patients, administration sharpened its focus on reducing our own ED diversion rates, length of stay, and the number of patients walking out without treatment and increasing patient satisfaction.

A management engineer with 30 years of experience brought his creativity to bear, working closely with us to use existing resources and talents to crank up the Healthcare Excellence Through Action Teams (HEAT). Members of ED and quality, finance, administration, lab, and radiology crafted the plan for active patient management. With 25% of hospital admissions coming through the ED, diversions and overcrowding had to be regarded as a hospital-wide issue rather than an ED problem. Patient holds in ED became known as "Parma Holds." Nurse managers on inpatient units signed an agreement with the ED to establish "hold beds" so patients could be moved promptly out of the ED. Lab and radiology committed to expediting ED orders. Physicians were asked to name another doctor to admit patients if they could not be reached.

A clinical supervisor for admitting, known as the "Bed Czar," was appointed to float between floors and keep admissions and discharges moving along to free up beds. This individual worked with admissions coordinators at area nursing homes to improve the flow of non-urgent nursing home patients. Admissions paperwork was transferred to the inpatient side, relieving ED staff. Bedside registration required a different triage process. Nursing managers assist the Bed Czar by notifying all nursing management staff

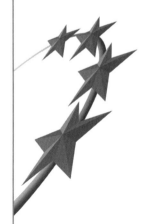

Parma Community General Hospital
Parma, Ohio

155

when ED is exceptionally full. Any nursing manager can call what is known as a "bed meeting," which briefly unites unit leaders to address the crisis and trigger movement of patients.

Within a year, diversion hours decreased by 33%. Parma Hospital's diversion hours dipped below 500 for the year, while hours of diversion continued to increase at all four other hospitals serving the western suburbs of Cuyahoga County. In fact, Parma Hospital's closest competitor had a 42% jump in diversion hours — more than 5,300 hours for the year.

We identified support RNs to provide clinical, emotional, and social support to patients and their families while in the ED. Support RNs are particularly attentive to patient needs; they recognize and can intercept potentially life-threatening conditions to ensure that patients receive immediate attention.

A new HealthMatics®ED computer helps us code patients as red, yellow, or green, based on acuity. Icons indicate which patients need lab work or X-rays and the system shows how long they've been in ED since registration. The system was modified to allow for real-time retrospective decision support.

As access improved, so did patient satisfaction. Satisfaction scores rose from the 21st to 68th percentile. Length-of-stay for treat-and-release patients fell 39.5%, to 2.48 hours from 4.1 hours a year earlier. The number of patients leaving without treatment or before being seen dropped 52%.

HEAT also spurred the opening of a six-bed subacute area with a dedicated physician. This is the first phase of a planned expansion that will nearly double the size of our emergency department. We need the additional space but we have demonstrated that we know how to work within constraints to improve the care and attention we give to all customers who are in need of our services.

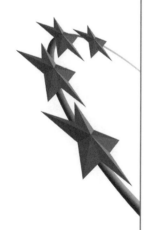

Parma
Community
General Hospital

Parma, Ohio

When the number of patients seeking care from an emergency department is twice what it was designed to handle, it is a problem. If, on top of physical constraints, inadequate staffing and inefficient processes are added, it is no wonder that patients become dissatisfied. Performance and process improvements—along with expansion and modernization of the facility—resulted in marked improvement in patient satisfaction and customer service when Lankenau Hospital initiated a comprehensive project to revitalize the emergency department and restore patient satisfaction.

Many patients and family members get their first impression of Lankenau Hospital through an emergency department encounter. Two major problems encumbered Lankenau's ED—overcrowding and an inadequate physical facility. Lankenau's ED was designed to handle 15,000 patients a year and was poorly equipped to accommodate the 30,000 patients seen annually. Several other significant issues needed attention: long delays, patient comfort and privacy, ambulance diversions, and adequate staffing. The ED staff and the medical staff also expressed frustration with these issues, which in turn diminished our ability to remain customer-focused.

Arduous planning and hard work created an ED with patient-friendly focus and efficient patient flow. Patient comfort and privacy were top priorities. A Fast Track unit was opened and a new, rapid triage system was instituted. An ED tracking system was installed. Decontamination equipment was obtained and staff was trained in disaster preparedness.

The physician staff committed to achieving excellence by conducting more thorough evaluations, ensuring definitive and ongoing management, improving documentation, and enhancing communication with attending physicians and residents. A comprehensive quality assurance was implemented with a focus on ED returns, radiographic discrepancies, transfer compliance, acute care denials, and mortality. Efforts to improve the management of acute ischemic stroke, myocardial infarction, and community-acquired pneumonia were coordinated with hospital committees.

A $9 million construction project began to transform the old ED, hidden in the rear of the hospital, into a new state-of-the-art facility located in the front of the institution. The new facility has increased capacity, universal function capability, and high-tech equipment. Emergency department staffing was augmented with new positions created, including nursing clinical leader, patient representative, inventory controller, and care manager. Physician coverage was increased and physician assistants added.

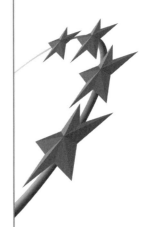

Lankenau Hospital

Lankenau, Pa.

Efficiency was enhanced by coordination with other departments: patient access (bedside registration); clinical lab (faxing lab results during computer down-time; specially marked bar code labels to designate ED specimens; facilitated lab ordering and result reporting); respiratory therapy (continuous nebulizer treatments); security (full-time ED security presence; patient visitation policy); radiology (filmless radiology system; diagnostic X-ray and CT scan facilities in ED; expanded radiology technologist coverage); transportation (dedicated ED transporter); and internal medicine (admission process, guidelines for the management of boarded patients, incorporated medical residents into ED "care team").

Hospital-wide changes now prevent ED overcrowding and diversions. New protocols define actions needed during pre-divert or diversion situations. Discharge processes were scrutinized for ways to expedite discharges. One solution was to create a discharge unit, where discharged patients are comfortably accommodated while awaiting transportation home. A new recruitment program attracts telemetry and emergency nurses. Long term strategic planning is developing more intensive care and telemetry beds, a medical short-stay unit, a rapid admission team, and new telemetry admission practices.

Overall patient satisfaction with emergency department service rose from 76.1 to 84.7, moving us from the 16th percentile to the 84th percentile in our peer group ranking. ED staff morale has dramatically improved; 20 of 21 questions were answered more favorably this year than last. ED visits increased 10% in the latest fiscal year and volume for the first three months of the current fiscal year is up 15%. Despite a surging census, divert hours have steadily declined, diminishing from 62 per month two years ago, to 48 per month last year, to 19 per month so far this year. Community confidence in Lankenau's ED has been restored, as indicated by our system's consumer-tracking surveys showing Lankenau ED is the first choice of 46% of the people in its service area, up from 35% six months earlier and 29% one year ago.

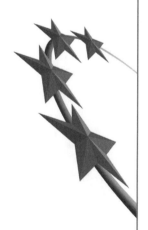

Lankenau
Hospital

Lankenau, Pa.

Six Sigma is one of the most talked-about systems for improving the quality of organizational processes. The Baldridge Criteria for Performance Excellence provides a systems-perspective for understanding performance management. Six Sigma methodologies and Baldridge award criteria helped an interdepartmental team at Robert Wood Johnson University Hospital at Hamilton isolate and remedy performance issues in the emergency department. These driving forces of change have resulted in sustained performance and satisfaction improvement. Patient satisfaction remains consistently above the 90th percentile and employee satisfaction was ranked in the 96th percentile after the most recent survey.

With a volume of approximately 50,000 annual visits, the ED at Robert Wood Johnson University Hospital at Hamilton is the point of entry for a majority of hospital admissions. An interdepartmental team led by the chief operating officer drives improvement efforts in the emergency department. Staff and physicians are involved in projects such as ED nurse-driven protocols, clinical pathways, and our automated documentation program.

We post a weekly patient satisfaction score dashboard with a traffic light indicator system (red, yellow, green) to quickly identify problem trends and to trigger rapid action-planning. We have an automated "Voice of the Customer" complaint management database from which complaints and compliments can be aggregated easily.

We have aligned performance incentives by combining both patient satisfaction and productivity measures in our compensation plan for our emergency physician partners. We now provide a quarterly bonus for employees based on the achievement of patient satisfaction targets.

Mobile cell phones are carried by all nurses and physicians in the department to enhance real-time information and rapid communication. Digital X-ray images in our picture archive and communication system are available to ED physicians and can be remotely accessed by attending physicians. We use an Ibex automated information and tracking system to reduce variance in the quality of our documentation.

Systems improvement was necessary before we could deliver on the bold promises of our service guarantee program. The "15/30" program states that patients will see a nurse within 15 minutes and a physician within 30 minutes or the ED visit is free. Within three months, we were able to reduce the average ED waiting time for admission by 25% using Six Sigma methodology. Nurse practitioners in PromptCare (fast-track) improved the timeliness of treatment initiation. We added a triage nurse and case management staff to our core staffing, and increased nurse-patient ratios to provide primary care.

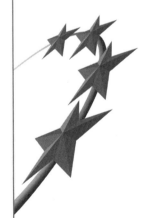

Robert Wood Johnson University Hospital at Hamilton

Hamilton, N.J.

Expanded physician hours improved "wait time to see physician" scores. Our goal is to achieve a benchmark target of 60 minutes for time held.

Two radiology suites now are physically located within the ED to reduce test turnaround time. Patient care representatives are stationed in the reception area, as well as the main ED, to welcome visitors and meet the needs of arriving patients.

A new state-of-the-art, 17,000-sq. ft. ED building accommodates a growing volume of 50,000 annual visits. All ED rooms are private with free TV service. We added a decontamination shower and serve as a regional center for emergency preparedness.

To reduce errors, we switched to an automated physician and nursing documentation system that virtually eliminated errors due to illegible transcription. It produces custom reports for performance improvement purposes. We use a Pyxis® drug dispensing system to safely administer medications.

Patient satisfaction scores in the 77th percentile initiated our resolve to improve performance. Results in patient satisfaction show a steady trend upward and remain consistently above the 90th percentile. Our latest employee satisfaction results reflect overall satisfaction in the 96th percentile. Most impressive were results in the areas of customer focus (99th percentile), satisfaction with senior leadership (98th percentile), recognition (91st percentile) and morale (91st percentile).

The hospital maintains the predominant position in the primary market, as measured by a survey of 500 community residents of Hamilton. Physicians rated our emergency services "significantly" higher than the database mean. We achieved excellence in clinical outcomes (PRO statewide recognition) with over 90% compliance in outcome indicators.

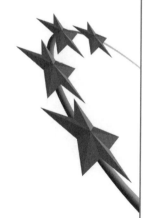

Robert Wood Johnson University Hospital at Hamilton

Hamilton, N.J.

Sophisticated methods of performance improvement occasionally uncover simple solutions. Duncan Regional Hospital installed digital clocks outside each exam room in the emergency department to remind otaff of tho lapcod timo cinco comoono lact intoractod with tho waiting patient. These clocks helped to narrow the distance between employees and customers after the hospital effectively tripled the square footage and doubled the capacity of the department to meet growing demand. This solution, combined with other changes, contributed to improving patient satisfaction. Nurses' attention to patients in the ED, as reported on satisfaction surveys, shot to the 95th percentile, up from the 34th percentile prior to the renovation.

Historically, Duncan Regional Hospital has been a high-performing hospital with patient satisfaction scores maintained consistently in the top 5% nationally over the last 12 years. We place great emphasis on the patient and family experience. We've gone through quality service training at the Disney Institute and built an entire guest services program around those principles.

Even with this emphasis, the emergency department presented a challenge. The ED ranked in the 55th percentile in overall patient satisfaction. We could rationalize why we were getting low scores; patients in rural settings are typically not accustomed to waiting. Most patients expect personalized, "one on one" care in an hour or less. The knee-jerk reaction was to add more staff to take care of increased patient load, but to add more caregivers wasn't an option given the realities of the Balanced Budget Act and significant nursing shortages.

When the emergency department was renovated, the number of exam rooms was expanded from 6 to 14. This tripled the square footage and doubled the capacity of the emergency department, which made it more challenging for employees to keep track of the "care and comfort" needs of patients who were waiting for tests or to see physicians.

Recognizing that busy staff does not perceive or experience time in the same way concerned patients do, we decided to install two digital clocks above the door of each room. One clock records the total amount of time a patient has been in the room; the second clock records the elapsed time since a patient had been checked on by a member of the hospital staff. This second clock is reset by team members each time they interact with the patient. The staff has the ability to see, at a glance, how long a particular patient had been in the ED, as well as how long it has been since someone on the staff communicated with them. The clocks also help physicians to prioritize their visits by looking to see who has been waiting for the longest period of time. The emergency department is staffed by trained volunteers who interface

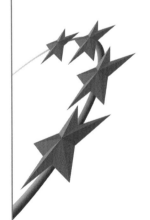

Duncan Regional Hospital

Duncan, Okla.

with patients and family members to keep them informed and to respond to requests for blankets, coffee and other needs.

The ED also took a look at how care was delivered and how technology and renovated space could help us expand our capabilities. We added a private triage area, automated medication dispensing system, and pneumatic transport tube system, all of which decreased turnaround times. The hospital contracted with a private, board-certified emergency physician group and hired physician assistants to expand services available. Televisions on articulated arms were added to every room to help take patients' minds off the wait time or their conditions. Wireless in-room registration was added, so patients went straight from triage into a room where registration information could be obtained while a nurse or doctor was taking care of them.

By systematically shifting our focus away from ourselves and toward patients and their families, we succeeded in increasing overall patient satisfaction for the emergency department. Keeping patients informed is just one of the reasons Duncan Regional Hospital's emergency department consistently achieves satisfaction scores ranked above the 90th percentile.

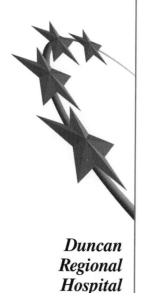

Duncan
Regional
Hospital

Duncan, Okla.

Emergency departments receive the entire continuum of patients seeking service – from drug addicts to trauma cases to children with the flu. Is the emergency department an appropriate place to co-mingle such a widely defined clientele? Prince William Hospital did not think so and ERjr was created to treat children with minor illnesses and injuries at times when pediatrician offices are closed. With four exam rooms, ERjr is staffed by a team of pediatricians and nurses dedicated to caring for children in a friendly environment, where Prince William staff can decrease the emotional impact of being in a hospital emergency room.

The service area population for Prince William Hospital is predominately young (average age 31.5 years), growing and middle/upper middle class. Our strategic plan identified that programs and services relating to women and children will continue to be volume drivers in our service area. ERjr has been a unique way for us to respond to the needs, preferences, and expectations of our market.

When the hospital conducted focus groups with members of the community, parents of children who had been seen recently in the emergency room identified a preference to have their children shielded from the crisis atmosphere of an adult emergency room. They also stated their preferences for a child-friendly environment that offered good clinical care, promptly delivered by nurses and physicians with special training in pediatrics. The medical director assembled a team of nurses, ancillary staff, and marketing staff to organize the program. It went from idea to implementation in six weeks.

ERjr is designed to offer all children (newborns to teenagers) immediate access to the special attention and compassionate care they need when pediatrician offices are closed. The location is separate from, but close to, the emergency room so registration remains at the ER.

Initially, the ERjr space was used by our occupational medicine department during the week. For weekends and evenings a pediatric cart was rolled into the department. Pictures were hung and pop-up toys appeared. The occupational medicine signs were covered by colorful ERjr signs. Not long after the program started, ERjr took over the entire area permanently. Now, the state-of-the-art equipment we use is tailor-made for children — from kid-sized blood pressure cuffs to casting supplies.

When Prince William Hospital opened ERjr we treated an average of 12 children daily in the ER. The hospital believed 23 patients a day was a realistic goal, given hours of operation, number of exam rooms, and staffing. In the past year, we treated as many as 50 children a day. For the last three months, the average intake of patients has been 35 a day. Physician offices are notified by ERjr staff when their patients are seen in the clinic.

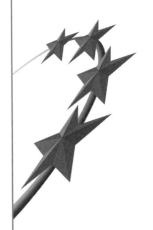

Prince William Hospital

Manassas, Va.

163

Our communications plan to promote the new service included an attractive logo and slogan — "We're here to make it all better" — used on all promotional materials. A local TV station featured ERjr on its 30-minute public affairs program. School groups regularly visit and tour the ERjr area.

The budget for ERjr was minimal, especially compared to the entire emergency department budget and other highly visible hospital projects such as our Birthing Center. There were no construction costs and few start-up expenses. We hired additional staff and spent $30,000 on the marketing campaign. This "patient-friendly" service in ERjr has generated positive word-of-mouth comments in the community. ERjr has been a good morale booster for the entire hospital.

Today, a child is typically in and out of ERjr in 67 minutes. We mail patient satisfaction surveys regularly and ask families to fill out exit evaluations as they leave. Patient satisfaction rose from 56% to 80% in the first six months and subsequently zoomed to 100%. ERjr has had a positive impact on the performance of the main emergency department, enabling it to focus on its specialized services for emergency and adult care. "Nurses overall quality of care" scores rose to 100% in the latest survey. Employee morale has risen along with the success.

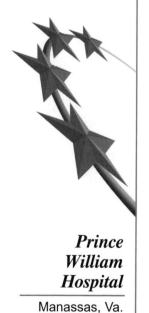

*Prince
William
Hospital*

Manassas, Va.

Fast Track is a program designed to speed medical services to patients who come to the emergency department with minor bumps, bruises, cuts, and colds. When patient dissatisfaction with service caused its ranking to drop from the 98th percentile to the 70th percentile, White County Medical Center's emergency department tackled one of the contributing causes. By implementing a Fast Track system to triage patients arriving at the ED on the weekends, length of stay for non-emergent patients was reduced 62%. This, along with other improvements, helped the department return to its previous level of performance.

Emergency room visits at White County Medical Center rose from 24,632 to 30,389 in three years, a 23% increase. During that same time, patient satisfaction scores dropped precipitously. Length of stay in the emergency room averaged 2.35 hours on weekends. We had to look for better way to respond to these patients.

After visiting emergency departments in other facilities and researching literature, a team composed of senior leadership and emergency department personnel determined that a Fast Track system in our emergency department was the optimal method to achieve improvement in declining patient satisfaction scores. Fast Track moves low-acuity patients out of the main flow of more serious medical cases and into a designated area of the emergency department. There, patients are treated and released from the hospital. Fast Track was initially opened on Saturdays to see non-emergent patients from 10 a.m. to 8 p.m., using two to three of our existing emergency rooms. Within five weeks, we extended its operation to Sundays. The only cost involved with the implementation of this program was related to bringing in an additional physician experienced in a family practice clinical environment to address non-emergent care concerns.

All patients entering the emergency department go through the triage process where the nurse assesses the patient. Patients referred to Fast Track are directed to a separate waiting area from those needing more emergent treatment. Average length of stay for those on Fast Track decreased to 53.6 minutes, a phenomenal 62% reduction. Reflecting the success of Fast Track and other performance improvement initiatives, patient satisfaction scores climbed and brought our ranking to the 94th percentile.

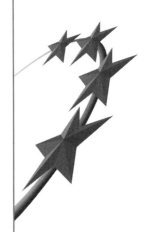

*White County
Medical Center*

Searcy, Ark.

As patient air transports increased, Indian Path Medical Center recognized the need for a clearly defined air transport process to better serve the community and to comply with regulations. A multidisciplinary team was created to decrease delays in patient air transport and improve safety. The team reviewed processes, developed procedures, and created a system for monitoring compliance. Since implementing the new procedures and training employees, Indian Path Medical Center now maintains 100% compliance with regulations.

Indian Path Medical Center, a member of Mountain States Health Alliance, is located in eastern Tennessee and is close to the Virginia and Kentucky state lines. Indian Path Medical Center receives patients from these three states, but we are not a trauma center. Patients experiencing trauma or life-threatening illnesses are transported to facilities better equipped to handle their needs by Mountain States Health Alliance's helicopter service, WINGS AIR RESCUE. As the number of transports increased, it became apparent that the process of patient air transport needed improvement.

A multidisciplinary team was chartered to review all transports to and from our medical center. We created flow charts of our processes, identified causes and effects, and streamlined new processes. By completing a simple "Air Transport Checklist" on every patient air transport, Indian Path Medical Center maintains 100% compliance with regulations. Using a newly created "Patient Air Transport" packet, all required documents are completed and signed. We renovated the helipad and added fixed lighting, a fire suppression system and a mounted storage cabinet to hold protective equipment, and other items. We defined roles, responsibilities, and accountabilities of staff and trained them about helicopter/helipad safety. Education included computer-based coursework to ensure competency.

Concurrent review of the transport by the house supervisor and retrospective review of the chart and checklist by the safety officer ensures our patient transport process is streamlined, efficient and safe for our staff and community.

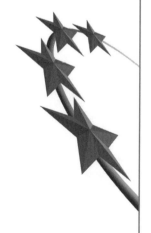

Mountain States Health Alliance

Johnson City, Tenn.

Smaller hospitals often deal with the problem of wasted food because of fluctuating patient census. An enterprising hospital director at Lindsborg Community Hospital came up with an idea to market home-styled meals to the public and created Healthy Fast Food to Go. Now, more than 600 nutritious meals each month are packaged by the dietary department and sold to the public. Food that previously would have been discarded now nourishes residents in the heartland of Kansas. The meal service also generates revenues that help to improve bottom line performance.

Most families find it difficult to determine how many to count on for dinner; try figuring out how many individuals are eating at a hospital on any given day. Lindsborg Community Hospital has 39 beds and serves an area population of 5,338. Our patient census fluctuates constantly, along with the number of staff and visitors that eat at the hospital. We might start the day with four patients and end the day with 12 or vice versa. With Meals on Wheels factored into the scenario, planning was very frustrating. Often, too much food was prepared which then had to be discarded.

Along came an innovative idea: Healthy Fast Food to Go. Home-cooked food from our hospital kitchen is now portioned into containers, quick-frozen while hot, sealed under clear plastic with a special machine and labeled with re-heating instructions. Meals are then frozen for sale to the general public. Our registered dietitian supervises the program and the meal preparation. The Healthy Fast Food to Go program has exceeded our expectations. It creates revenue and reduces waste. More importantly, the food is tasty, healthy, and convenient.

Currently the kitchen sells more than 600 frozen meals a month. Some customers purchase the meals because of diet restrictions, others for convenience, but all return for more because they're delicious. To begin this innovative program we purchased a $1,000 sealing machine and hoped it would pay for itself in a year's time. It took only four months to recoup the cost of the sealing machine.

Each meal contains about 300 calories and is suitable for people on special diets. The recipes are low-fat, with no additional sugar or salt. All meals are complete with meat, vegetable and a side dish. Here is a sampling of what $2.75 will buy: 1) turkey breast with real mashed potatoes and gravy, and green beans; 2) chicken and noodles, peas, and applesauce; or 3) swiss steak, baked potato, and mixed vegetables. Meals can be heated in a microwave or conventional oven. This program fills a niche for people who are not homebound and therefore do not qualify for our Meals on Wheels program. The meals fill a void in our community not only for those who find it difficult to get out, but also those who are "cooking challenged," college students and singles who dislike cooking for themselves.

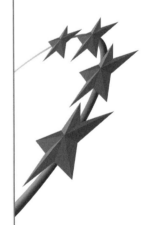

Lindsborg
Community
Hospital

Lindsborg, Kan.

Success of the program can be evidenced in the number of meals sold. The first month we packaged meals for sale, we sold 17 meals; the number soon rose to 92 meals and by the third month we delivered 392 frozen meals. The numbers now hold fairly steady, averaging more than 600 meals a month.

It costs approximately 25 cents per meal for packaging materials and $1.25 per meal for food contents. This leaves $1.25 profit from each meal sold. Last year, we sold 5,963 meals and generated $17,152 in revenue.

Healthy Fast Food to Go is taken very seriously by the hospital dietary staff. They view the project as a means of helping the general public, reducing waste, and producing revenue for the hospital. The dietary staff has many years of experience cooking for this predominately Swedish community. They know what the public likes and, more importantly, what the community needs to be eating. The staff uses this knowledge to creatively package foods that will appeal to our population. From trying new recipes, packaging the meals, taking orders, and selling meals, everyone has a part.

Our patrons may be single, widowed, or married, young or old, healthy or diabetic. But one thing is constant…our meals fill a void in our community and beyond. One of our regular customers drives 140 miles round trip every six to eight weeks to purchase 40 meals for her elderly father. Over the past four years, she has tried other options because it takes four hours out of her day to pick the meals up, but her father has not liked the taste of other alternatives.

Similarly, 350 meals are purchased every month by a community agency working with persons with developmental disabilities. The balance are sold primarily to elderly individuals in the community. Another benefit of the meal program is that nursing staff is able to offer a patient an appetizing hot meal after the kitchen has closed.

Lindsborg Community Hospital's mission states, "Partners caring for the health of the Smoky Valley community." Our mission is our passion. The Healthy Fast Food to Go program is an innovative way of helping people maintain their independence by providing quick, healthy, and delicious meals.

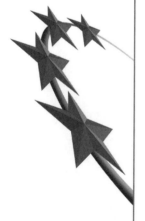

Lindsborg Community Hospital

Lindsborg, Kan.

The hospital cafeteria gives employees a place to go to enjoy a brief respite from their busy work. It is also the destination to which many family members retreat when they need a break. The new CrossRoads Café at Conemaugh Memorial Medical Center offers customers what they seek: ambiance, extended hours of operation and convenient food preparation sites that serve delicious, healthy food selections. What is even more impressive is the 50% growth in retail sales since the new facility opened. Profitable performance and customer satisfaction combined with revenue growth made the CrossRoads Café a wise investment, as well as a popular destination.

Before the opening of CrossRoads Café, employees and visitors to Conemaugh Memorial Medical Center had limited choices when it came to mealtime. They could go to the main cafeteria area, an antiquated facility built in the mid-1940s, to get customary hospital fare from the traditional hospital cafeteria line or they could visit a second cafeteria at the other end of the campus in a building acquired as part of a merger with a nearby hospital. Hours of operation at both of those sites were restricted to two hours around each mealtime. A small grill/café area that featured a limited choice of sandwich selections and vending machines offered employees their only other food and drink alternatives.

Our vision to consolidate the separate cafeterias into a state-of-the-art facility required careful planning and we relied heavily on the experts – our employees. We could not ignore the fact that they had good ideas that would make the new operation more pleasurable and convenient for guests and staff. Training also was important to ensure the success of this new venture. The facility had a new layout and featured new equipment and processes. Employees understood early on that not only would they be trained, but management would work along side them to make sure we all thrived as a team during this transition.

After all the planning, training, and hard work, we opened our new café and received rave reviews. The CrossRoads Café is an innovative facility that offers numerous food selection sites including: deli, grill, pizza/pasta station, beverage area, salad bar, and dessert locations. The salad bar is more than twice the size of the one in the old location and features several specialty salads and healthy choices daily. For anyone wanting the "traditional" hot meal, our Chefs Feature area is available. The food there has been enhanced to include not only traditional items, but also healthy choice, low-fat, "wellness" selections.

Several touch screen stations are available for guests to easily order meals. Food is produced on demand; when an order is placed, that meal is prepared. As the orders become available, those numbers scroll across screens located throughout the service area so guests don't have to stand in front of the food

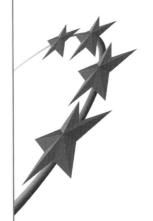

*Conemaugh
Memorial
Medical Center*

Johnstown, Pa.

preparation area. If they do prefer to wait at the station, we provide breaking news broadcasts on the touch screens. Check-out is no longer an issue. Four registers are operational at main meal times. Debit cards are available and frequently have been purchased and given as gifts.

Location is no longer an issue. Our Crossroads Café is at the cross roads of our facility. The central location allows easy access from inpatient units and outpatient departments alike. A winding tile pattern on the floor creates the impression of a narrow road and small café tables are situated on either side. The main dining area is constructed of oak, glass, and green/brown upholstery, providing an "outdoor" ambiance with rich earth-tones. Hours of operation allow dining from 6 a.m. until 10:30 p.m. A new vending area offers full-meal selections, as well as traditional "grab-n-go" items when café service is suspended. Lighting fixtures provide a soft white light to accent the natural lighting from two external walls of windows.

We planned a spacious area for a new gift shop run by our auxiliary. There is space to offer a wide selection of gift items, flowers, balloons, and novelties. Beautiful glass display cases line our streetscape, giving the impression of a small Italian piazza; a restaurant is on one side and a quaint shopping area is on the other.

Speaking of new ideas, a brand new concept for this facility was the Gourmet Bean beverage kiosk. The made-to-order milkshakes have been a huge hit, as have specialty coffees. Homemade specialty desserts are available at this location for those with an insatiable sweet tooth.

It is clear that involving employees in decisions and investing in their development has done much to build employee confidence and satisfaction. Internal customer (employee) satisfaction has gone from the 6th percentile to the 80th percentile in a period of two years. In addition to the improvements in employee satisfaction, we've also experienced notable improvements in customer satisfaction. During the past six months there has been a 20% increase in satisfaction in our customer base. We're demonstrating top line revenue results, as well. Total sales have increased by 50% over the past two years, which translates to $455,000. Projected sales for the coming year are an additional $300,000. Sales for the Gourmet Bean kiosk generated $150,000 in the first year of operation.

Our efforts have contributed substantially to the financial performance of our operation and more importantly, to the satisfaction of our external and internal customers.

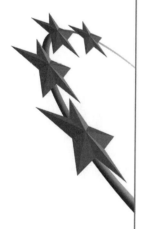

Conemaugh
Memorial
Medical Center

Johnstown, Pa.

170

Food service is typically delivered on a pre-determined schedule and without regard for customer preferences. Yet, it is widely accepted that the patient's ability to exercise some measures of control and choice contributes positively to the patient experience. Hamot Medical Center transformed meal service experiences when the room service dining program was launched. Patients now order meals from an expanded menu and the food is delivered to them. Since the program began, food waste has decreased, the number of guests ordering room service has increased from 20 meals to 500 meals a month, and satisfaction with food service now ranks in the 90th percentile or better.

Hamot Medical Center relies on patient satisfaction feedback to fuel our pursuit of service excellence. Our goal has been to achieve and sustain improved patient satisfaction ratings for meal service. Based on monthly and quarterly satisfaction reports, we implemented various efforts that resulted in temporary successes. However, patient perceptions of the overall quality of meals continued to fall short of expectations. In an attempt to become more patient-centric, Hamot introduced At Your Request™ as an innovative approach to achieving service excellence.

Our room service dining program offers a pleasant alternative to traditional meal service by permitting patients to order meals as they would in a hotel. Patients phone in their meal request when they are hungry and their food is delivered to their rooms within 45 minutes or less. Replacing the inflexible delivery of meals at three specified times throughout the day, the system adapts to the patient's preferences and his/her desired schedule of eating. A restaurant-style menu offers variety to please every patient's taste. As a service enhancement, visiting family members and friends may also place orders from the menu and remain in the patient's room to dine.

When placing an order, the patient dials the menu line and speaks directly with a nutrition technician. This employee greets the patient, receives the meal request, and inputs the order into a computerized order-entry system. If the patient's menu selection fails to meet dietary restrictions, the nutrition technician immediately helps the patient make an alternate choice. The order is electronically forwarded to the kitchen and the meal is prepared and delivered to the patient's room. If a patient fails to place an order by a designated time, the computer system alerts the nutrition technician to contact the patient. For patients unable to place orders for themselves, numerous options exist, including personal assistance, family assistance, or in some cases, automatic selection of nutritious meals.

To avoid placing additional responsibility on the nursing staff, the nutrition department created the position of Room Service Ambassador. The ambassador meets with new admissions to ensure each patient understands

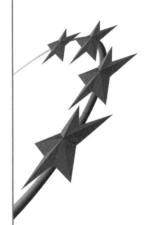

Hamot
Medical
Center

Erie, Pa.

how to order meals. The Room Service Ambassador provides timely response to dietary questions as they arise, intervenes to minimize nursing involvement in meal-related issues, and provides immediate service recovery, when necessary. The ambassador can distribute basic nutritional information to patients, and assist those in need with referrals to the staff dietitians. Newspapers are available to be delivered with patient meals, at their request.

As with any new program, we faced expected and unexpected challenges. Initially, there was resistance to the system change until everyone became more comfortable and familiar with the process. The census created an unexpected test. The historical census data on which patient demand was based proved to be an inaccurate estimate of the staff and service capabilities needed. Throughout the first months of the program's implementation, Hamot actually experienced unusually high patient volumes. We worked these issues out and At Your Request™ has proven to be a huge success. Hamot's patient satisfaction ratings have soared through the roof.

Hamot Medical Center has distinguished itself from its peers of similar size by advancing from the 44th to the 95th percentile in areas relating to the quality, temperature, courtesy of delivery and overall satisfaction with food service. In comparison to other 100 top hospitals, room service boosted Hamot's food service performance ahead of 99% of the best facilities in the nation.

In addition to improving patient satisfaction with meals, Hamot is beginning to experience additional benefits of the program. Because patients order what they want, when they want, At Your Request™ dining has reduced food waste. The notable improvements in food appearance, variety, and quality have also resulted in a significant increase in the number of guest tray orders. In contrast to serving approximately 20 guest trays each month prior to room service, an estimated 400 to 500 visitors a month now take advantage of this hotel-style amenity.

Patients are thrilled with the personalized service we offer. Rave reviews from the organization's top food critics have become the norm in monthly comment reports. Hamot's room service dining is just one of the organization's many innovative approaches to focus on the patient and provide the best quality care and service.

Hamot has experienced improved satisfaction ratings over the last four quarters, and the most recent monthly report indicates a continuation of this trend. Comments provided by patients offer additional indications of the program's lasting success.

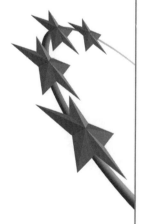

Hamot
Medical
Center

Erie, Pa.

Improving patient satisfaction can be as basic as providing individualized meals delivered by friendly and helpful employees. Yet, given the complex processes that are involved in preparing and serving meal selections, as ordered by the patient from a limited menu and at the right temperatures, it is no small feat to offer an expanded menu and institute hotel-like room service in a hospital. The Nebraska Medical Center's room service program allows patients to order meal selections when they are hungry or in the mood to eat. The meals are often delivered within 30 minutes. As a result, patient satisfaction increased 15%.

The array of entrées offered on the room service menu at The Nebraska Medical Center is diverse and patients are able to order their selections the way they like them and when they want them. To accommodate this program, our kitchen went through several modifications. Previously, the kitchen was set up for quantity cooking with foods prepared and held in warmers until time of service. Our cooks now prepare food to order and the tray line has disappeared.

Our system is designed for a 45-minute turnaround from the time that the patient places a meal order to the time that order is received. We've managed to consistently exceed this performance benchmark, to as low as an average time of 32 minutes in some months. The diet office staff takes telephone orders quickly and establishes rapport with the patients. Our room service attendants, who deliver the made-to-order meals, also are able to develop relationships with the patients.

Trays are carefully checked to guarantee accuracy before the tray is delivered. All interactions are scripted to assure consistency and thoroughness during the order and delivery processes. The taste, temperature and attractive presentation of the food, combined with the convenience of ordering from an expanded menu and interacting with friendly employees, create lasting, positive impressions.

The computer program used by the diet office staff is programmed to make sure the foods patients order are consistent with their dietary restrictions. Currently, our hours of operation are from 6:30 a.m. to 6:30 p.m., but we anticipate expanding these hours to create even greater flexibility in meeting patients' needs and preferences.

Since instituting the program, our patient satisfaction scores have improved by 15%. On any given day, 70% of the patients at our 735-licensed bed hospital receive their meals through room service. Our responsiveness to meet patients' needs and hopes for delicious meals on their schedule, not ours, demonstrates the commitment of food and nutritional services department to deliver extraordinary customer service.

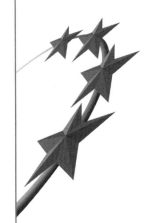

The Nebraska Medical Center

Omaha, Neb.

Performance Improvement
Nourishing Patients with Special Needs

The prevalence of lactose intolerance and diabetes is very high in Hispanic and Asian populations. Many of the customers served by Garden Grove Hospital are of these ethnic origins and consumption of dietary products is problematic. They seldom tolerate full liquid diets. To anticipate and address the special needs of patients, the Food and Nutrition Services Team initiated the Full Liquid Diet Deletion Project. The project decreased the number of full liquid diets ordered by physicians to less than 0.5% of all diet orders.

Many customers of Garden Grove Hospital are lactose intolerant and unable to consume full liquid diets. Physicians who routinely order full liquid diets for their patients often are not aware of the complications inherent in the diet. High protein/high calorie clear liquid supplements or soft/regular diets can be tolerated without adverse consequence by patients in most instances, but many physicians are unaware of these options. Given the high percentage of patients who cannot tolerate liquid diets, we were aware of the necessity to educate physicians and nurses about full liquid diets and options.

Early intervention is the key to providing uninterrupted service to patients and averting problems. When a full liquid diet is ordered for a patient with lactose intolerance, a personal nutrition attendant phones the nursing unit to suggest alternatives and asks nursing staff to discuss the matter with the physician. In most cases, this proactive step of alerting the nursing staff results in revisions to the diet orders before the next meal service. The optimal solution, however, was to consult with nursing and medical staff to inform them of options and help them anticipate the nutritional restrictions and special needs of some patients.

For six months prior to implementation of the Full Liquid Diet Deletion Project, full liquid diets averaged 4% of all diet orders. Six months after we began our educational efforts, full liquid diets decreased to less than 0.5%. Patient satisfaction also improved as the appropriateness of dietary orders was anticipated.

Our efforts to discourage full liquid diet orders have paid off. Our initiative also has had a wider impact. As word of our initiative spread, other hospitals contacted us. We established a policy and procedure, "Nutrition: Patient Meal Service and Food Texture Progression," that addresses the deletion of the full liquid diet. With the support of our nursing and physician colleagues, we have been able to nourish and satisfy patients with special needs.

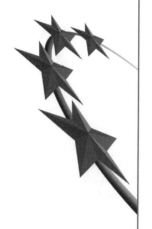

Garden Grove Hospital

Garden Grove, Calif.

174

Despite difficulties in stanching operational losses, employee defections, and customer dissatisfaction, some organizations continue to operate departments in the red because they don't want to introduce "outsiders" into the family. Yet, as The Queen's Medical Center discovered, once inside, a company providing management services can quickly become a valued member of the team by performing to exceed expectations. Since outsourcing the management of the food and nutrition department, sales have doubled, employee satisfaction has improved 33%, and $1.7 million has been saved as a result of the investment in the relationship.

The Queen's Medical Center previously maintained its own staff and management for preparation of patient meals, cafeteria service, and catering. For a number of reasons, we decided to outsource the management of the food & nutrition division. The first order of business was to renovate the dining room and add new kitchen equipment. A "ServSave" system has been installed, which helps decrease food waste and overproduction. The department went from a decentralized cook freeze, patient tray delivery system to a centralized cook and chill system. These changes allowed the department to increase productivity by 50%, change the skill mix of employees and at the same time, increase the patient food quality and satisfaction.

The menu was completely revamped and now features food items that have added extra value and a flare not typically found in a hospital setting. The new team contracted with a local restaurant chef to help develop menu items and prepare a special entrée once a month. Other improvements include a Starbucks coffee cart and the addition of two mobile food carts to serve hospital employees who are constantly on the go and often unable to take time for a meal in the cafeteria.

We have calculated that the new management company has saved the medical center $1.7 million. Food and nutrition department sales in have increased from $1.2 million a year to $2.3 million. Quality, variety, and value have increased. Food service employee satisfaction has gone up 33%. Customer satisfaction has improved 34%. These benefits, along with the financial savings, have contributed to the value of the relationship.

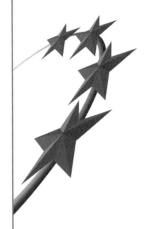

*The Queen's
Medical Center*

Honolulu, Hawaii

Tight controls on inventory help health care organizations manage costs, improve productivity, and avoid service breakdowns. With the help of one of its suppliers, Vernon Manor developed an inventory control system that accurately tracks supplies and gives timely information to departments when replenishments are needed. The new procedures have helped to reduce mysterious disappearances of costly supplies. The system has saved money and improved employee satisfaction.

Vernon Manor implemented an inventory control system with the assistance of a medical supply vendor. By using creative ideas and suggestions from employees within the organization, the inventory is now up to date and as cost-effective as ever.

Our tracking system for the volume and frequency of restocked items identifies consumption patterns that may exceed the norm. For example, we noticed we were reordering washcloths and face towels at a much higher rate than previously. One of our employees, a laundry attendant, suggested that we stamp the name of our nursing home on each wash cloth. This identifying mark discourages people from removing the wash cloths from the facility. Because our housekeeping department now monitors how many wash clothes go to each unit and how many are returned to the laundry, employees are more careful not to throw linens away. When the numbers come up short, the housekeeping department is notified to inspect the garbage. The savings to date from this new procedure has been $600 in three months.

We also created a supply room for each of our four resident units. These are stocked with a set number of supplies, such as paper products and adult diapers, and they are replenished twice a day. Any changes to the usual and customary levels of inventories maintained triggers an inquiry to identify the cause and it helps us to make adjustments. Our monitoring system has enabled us to generate cost savings while ensuring staff has the supplies they need to accommodate the residents' needs. We have worked diligently to decrease costs of doing business during these tough times and are making progress.

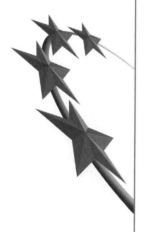

Vernon Manor

Vernon, Conn.

Mayo Clinic in Scottsdale tackled problems created by inefficient billing, confusing bills and patient dissatisfaction when it undertook a major conversion of the billing system. The patient financial services department anticipated one of the most important aspects of any major change initiative: communication. By keeping everyone informed about the status of the conversion while this technical project was implemented over a period of 3½ years, Mayo Clinic in Scottsdale kept internal and external customers happy.

D uring a period of years, patient and employee dissatisfaction with Mayo Clinic in Scottsdale's (MCS) billing system became more and more pronounced. Our employees experienced frustration with operational inefficiencies. We also had difficulty helping patients understand their bills. During focus groups, patients told us that our bills were confusing. They wanted an easier-to-read format and detailed information about services and charges. Administration fully supported the decision to increase patient and employee satisfaction by converting to a new billing system that would be shared with Mayo Clinic in Rochester, Minn., (MCR).

A Project Team, comprised of employees from multiple areas within MCS and MCR, was responsible for installing a system designed to generate a consolidated clinic and hospital bill and an itemized statement of charges. A Service Team was formed to identify and resolve internal and external customer service issues. Managers of the patient financial services department (PFS) solicited and shared employee feedback with the Service Team, which was used to develop a communications plan to keep PFS's customers – employees, physicians, payers, vendors, Medicare officials, government leaders and patients apprised of the project's status.

Expectations and enthusiasm for the project were so high that the Service Team had to clarify that the new system would not eliminate third-party payers or cause patients to like the bills any better. The team issued a statement identifying that the project goals were to: 1) create a new bill format that would be easier for patients to understand and 2) make information and support resources available pre- and post-conversion.

We expected PFS employees who were already proficient with the existing billing system to be anxious about learning a new system. Prior to the conversion, PFS employees attended classes on coping with organizational change. They learned about the new billing system by attending educational sessions scheduled throughout the year before the conversion. We used monthly newsletters, e-mail news flashes and presentations at management, departmental, and committee meetings to prepare everyone in the organization for the coming changes.

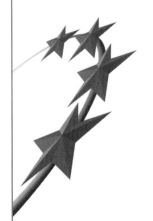

*Mayo Clinic
in Scottsdale*

Scottsdale, Ariz.

It was necessary to educate patients also. The team oversaw the design of a consumer-oriented Web page and a Web site for physicians to reference. A CD with information about billing was created. Patient education classes about general and Medicare billing were scheduled. The team also developed two new patient brochures, *Mayo Billing and You* and *Mayo Medicare and You.* An area near registration was renovated to provide a confidential setting for patients with billing questions. Before conversion, a sample of the new bill and itemized statement was mailed, with a cover letter from MCS administration, to 58,000 patients with active accounts.

Because Mayo Clinic Hospital expected to experience 24 hours of system downtime during conversion, the Service Team prepared clinical managers for this event. Presentations began months ahead to communicate progress on the conversion and how it would affect patient care units. We prepared samples of new statements to use as teaching tools and alerted managers to questions that they might be asked.

The Service Team received praise for its role in preparing the hospital for downtime. A representative comment written on the post-conversion survey stated, "All in all, the downtime at the hospital was well planned and executed. Issues were minor and this was a true example of excellent teamwork."

Patients were well-informed and their expectations were managed for the duration of this project. Before the conversion, satisfaction with the services provided by PFS improved 20% from our efforts to be more responsive to patient needs and expectations. Since the time of the conversion, patient satisfaction has increased an additional 14%. Patient satisfaction with billing and customer service continues to improve.

The number and nature of patient calls received by the PFS Call Center indicate satisfaction with the new bill format and itemized statement of charges. Immediately after conversion, fewer than 2% of calls were related to not understanding the new bill. A major change inevitably generates confusion and questions, but the number of calls received by the call center, which averages 375 to 400 a day, remained relatively constant for two months after conversion because patients were well informed and they anticipated the changes.

Just two months before the billing system conversion, PFS employee satisfaction was measured at its highest level ever. Employees looked forward to a new system that would make their jobs easier.

Despite a three-year project timeline, the commitment of the Project Team during this billing system conversion was unwavering. Members carried out their responsibilities with enthusiasm. Maintaining cohesion among team members separated by 1,500 miles, for three years, required creativity and dedication to achieving our common goals.

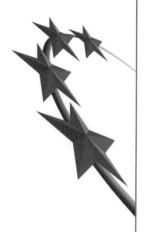

***Mayo Clinic
in Scottsdale***

Scottsdale, Ariz.

In an effort to improve the care of terminally-ill patients, health care institutions are using evidenced-based approaches to construct more positive methods for supporting dying patients and their family members. Daniel Freeman Memorial Hospital used a multidisciplinary approach to develop clinical pathways, education, and implementation guidelines that encourage all members of the patient care team to help patients transition from life in a manner that protects their rights, promotes their well being, and supports their loved ones. One year later, code status at the time of death doubled, and repetitive, invasive procedures used on "no code" patients declined by up to 63%.

Life is a gift from God that is to be cherished and respected in all its stages. This philosophy is embraced by the Sisters of St. Joseph of Carondelet and Daniel Freeman Memorial Hospital. Nurses, physicians and staff from departments such as pharmacy, social services, and volunteer services assembled to form a Comfort Care Team. We met to discuss end-of-life care and review how current practices met the tenets of the mission and philosophy of our hospital.

Using our performance improvement (PI) model, the Comfort Care Team assessed the current knowledge in this practice area and explored evidence-based literature on care for the dying. The team focused on developing a model that would help terminal patients transition from life in a manner that protects their rights, promotes their well being, supports their loved ones, and encourages all members of the patient care team to participate in their care.

The team conducted a baseline chart review to identify the population and look at ways to objectively measure behaviors that demonstrate use of comfort care. The team reviewed the charts of 42 patients who died at the facility. The deaths were considered expected, with diagnoses such as terminal cancer, multi-system failure, and end-stage organ disease. We reviewed the following indicators: code status at time of death; documentation of a futility note (i.e., "further care is futile, there is nothing else to be done"); documentation of a "good death;" and use of invasive procedures on no code patients. These data served as a baseline measure of the practice patterns at the hospital. We also conducted staff interviews to assess their level of comfort in caring for dying patients and what they perceived to be educational needs.

Based on review of the literature and existing models of comfort/palliative care, we developed a three-phase action plan that defined the Comfort Care process. The initial phase involved developing a clinical pathway (a multidisciplinary plan of care), producing preprinted orders for symptom management (with suggested assessments, treatments, and pharmacologic and non-pharmacologic interventions) and creating a medication guidelines reference. All three documents were thoroughly reviewed and approved by all appropriate medical staff committees.

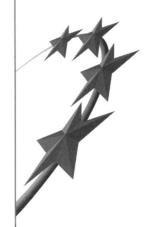

Daniel Freeman Memorial Hospital

Inglewood, Calif.

During the second phase of the process, a subgroup of resource personnel conducted in-service education for the staff of nursing units, medical staff committees and ancillary departments. The training emphasized the needs of a dying patient and family and the appropriate use of physical, psychologic, spiritual, cultural, and emotional interventions to ease transition through the dying process.

Implementation was achieved in the final phase. We initiated a house-wide poster campaign, conducted a seminar for community members on the Comfort Care process and provided continuing education for nursing home administrators and dialysis center personnel. The goal was to familiarize as many people and disciplines as possible about Comfort Care and to encourage their support.

The Comfort Care process has evolved over time. The medication guideline proved to be an invaluable tool because it empowered staff to collaboratively approach physicians about improved symptom management. Ongoing education continues to assist staff in developing their own level of comfort and expertise in this process.

The Comfort Care Team conducted a one year post-implementation chart review on 50 patients meeting the same initial criteria. Our goal was to evaluate the impact of the program. Our review revealed that No Code status increased from 24% to 50%; Futility Note and No Code status increased from 25% to 57%; documentation of Good Death increased from 23% to 40%. The use of mechanical ventilators decreased from 31% to 18%; blood transfusions decreased from 31% to 18% and repetitive labs decreased from 63% to 46%.

These data support an objective measure of behavioral change reflecting the appropriate use of Comfort Care. Anecdotal case reports also demonstrate improved staff and family satisfaction with the use of this process.

There is still much work to be done to promote the Comfort Care process and effect necessary changes to meet the needs of all who are involved in end-of-life care. By supporting this process, the organization actively demonstrates commitment to our mission and philosophy to cherish and respect life "from conception through death to life eternal."

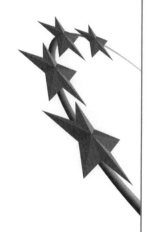

**Daniel Freeman
Memorial Hospital**

Inglewood, Calif.

Although the word "peaceful" is sometimes used to describe end-of-life experiences, all too often, anguish and pain are terms attributed to the process of dying. Treatment that enhances comfort and support can be provided when the dying person, primary caregivers, physicians, and staff agree on how care will be administered. Palliative care continues to be woven into the fabric of St. John's Regional Medical Center, and its innovative end-of-life care program is designed to build these mechanisms of support. Although financial considerations are secondary, St. John's has been able to identify a cost savings of $1 million as a result of the palliative care provided to over 700 patients.

St. John's Regional Medical Center is a mission-driven organization with a culture steeped in collaboration, innovation, and excellence. This culture, coupled with support from all levels within the organization, nurtured the development of a patient centered, end-of-life care program designed to improve the way patients die in our facility and to support their families during that difficult time. Our Palliative Care program flows from our mission and values that uphold the dignity of all persons and reverence for life in all its stages. Financial savings are secondary, but they reflect our value of integrity that holds us to wise use of human and fiscal resources.

Our vision was to create a healing place – in our hospital, in nursing facilities, and within our community. We define healing as "promotion of hope and prevention of despair for those experiencing terminal illness." We have designed a comprehensive model for supportive care of the dying, their families, and the community.

Today, our three-bed unit provides a home-like environment for patients and families where they can experience the final phase of life with support for their spiritual, emotional, and physical needs. The service is driven by the needs and preferences of the patient and family. Our model uses an interdisciplinary team approach led by a palliative care coordinator. Patient average length of stay is three days with our longest stay being 17 days. Eighty percent of our patients die while in the program, but 20% are discharged, most of them to home with hospice services or to long term care facilities.

Some organizations are reluctant to provide in-house palliative care, concerned that the program will increase expenses. A simple comparison of the costs of critical care and non-critical care rooms identifies the potential to save money. We developed other models to further demonstrate how respecting patient and family wishes enables us to be good stewards of our resources.

We used several methods to track cost-savings. Our first attempt to track savings was to look at the cost of rooms. A critical care room costs twice as much as a non-critical care room. Therefore, if a patient was transferred

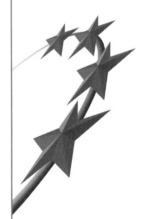

St. John's Regional Medical Center

Joplin, Mo.

from critical care to hospice care, money was saved. Obtaining estimates of direct costs was a little more challenging. A review of our palliative care and financial databases allowed us to capture room rates, cost of procedures, pharmaceuticals, and supplies and to project savings. Because there can be large variations in cost per patient day, especially in critical care, the most accurate method of determining cost savings is to directly examine each individual patient's cost before and after entering the end-of-life program. The average cost per patient per day can then be calculated before and after entering this palliative care program. The value of this method is that it is definitive, although it is too labor intensive for routine use. Regardless of which method we used, we consistently demonstrated direct cost savings.

We believe in the value of this ministry to the dying and their families and to the hospital. Based on pre- and post- data, satisfaction and financial cost savings were significantly increased after opening the unit.

Medical staff referrals and support for the program have been tremendous, with 97% of referring physicians using standing orders. In satisfaction surveys of bereaved family members, 97% state that their loved one's pain was controlled "well" or "very well." The overall satisfaction rating for the program is 4.9 on a 5-point scale. We've seen a 35% increase in organ and tissue donations in the past two years. Donations to our program have increased, from $400 a year to $14,844 two years later and typically arrive with expressions such as, "This was so wonderful for us; we want it to be there for others when they need it." Cards and letters from families are extremely affirming.

In 2004, the American Hospital Association bestowed upon us one of their most prestigious awards, the Circle of Life Citation of Honor. This award recognizes innovative palliative care/end-of-life programs.

St. John's Regional Medical Center's model of end-of-life care, in conjunction with financial tracking, demonstrates that it is possible to provide excellent physical, emotional and spiritual care to dying patients and their families with minimal expense and significant cost savings to the institution.

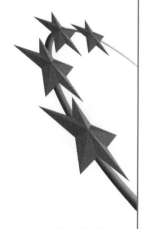

St. John's
Regional
Medical Center

Joplin, Mo.

CHAPTER 7
LEARNING & LEADERSHIP

—— LEARNING & LEADERSHIP ———————

Hospitals that rely on market or satisfaction research to broadcast the voice of the customer rarely understand their customers the way market leaders do. Bristol Hospital's success as a leader in building and sustaining customer and employee satisfaction is due, in great part, to its commitment to listen and hear what customers and employees have to say. The Patient Partners program gives management and staff opportunities to gain unique perspectives on customer expectations.

Bristol Hospital monitors patient perceptions and builds personal relationships with patients, families and other customers through our Patient Partners program. Patient Partners are given patient assignments and become each patient's partner and personal advocate. They help patients navigate the system and determine how we can proactively respond to their unique personal needs and exceed their expectations. Patient Partners visit their assigned patients daily during their hospital stay and maintain contact with them after they are discharged. Patient Partners continue this relationship with the patient for "life." If the patient returns to our hospital, the same partner is paired with that patient, whenever possible. If a patient has had a particularly rocky service history, the Patient Partner can interpret that patient's special needs or circumstances to staff.

Our Patient Partners are "in touch" with patients and families and they relay information so we can monitor trends and issues. We can then alert leaders in specific areas when we fall short of our goals so recovery can be initiated.

Bristol Hospital has a patient survey response rate of close to 40% and we monitor customer satisfaction on a daily basis. Customer surveys and comments are forwarded to department managers who are expected to call patients who rate performance as "poor" or "very poor" on any related dimension of service. Raw score results and percentile ranks are reported on a monthly basis so everyone is aware of where they stand in regard to patient satisfaction.

Bristol Hospital is just as diligent about staying close to employees. To "take the pulse" of the organizational psyche, we administer "Your Line" employee feedback surveys 6 to 8 times a year. These mini-surveys ask employees to share their opinions about a variety of issues; from physical plant changes to how prepared they feel in their jobs. Results are reported to senior management and then back to the employees. Our leadership team rounds and is clearly visible. Members frequently engage employees in informal discussions so they hear the voice of the workforce without distortion or interruption.

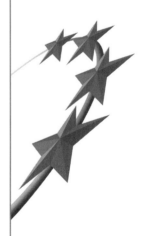

*Bristol
Hospital*

Bristol, Conn.

Whether a person interacts directly with patients or works behind the scenes to enhance patient care, Bristol Hospital has the means to recognize staff in a number of ways. Employees who have been named positively in a patient survey, letter, or telephone call appear on a Wall of Fame. We have a WOW Hotline and WOW certificates, which enable peers to recognize staff. The WOW program also feeds into an awards program that was instituted to recognize employees who demonstrate commitment to our organizational values.

Bristol Hospital reinvests financial success back into the workforce. A monetary bonus for all employees is distributed when patient satisfaction goals are attained. We hold frequent celebrations and "thank you" events for milestones of achievement such as sustaining service excellence, JCAHO accreditation, and successful capital campaigns.

In these ways and many others, Bristol Hospital maintains the proximity and perspective to make strategic decisions and operational improvements that respond to patient and employee needs and expectations.

We realize the strong correlation between employee and patient satisfaction, and the power of word-of-mouth advertising and internal marketing. We relentlessly pursue our customer relationship strategy, embracing our primary customers—patients, employees, and community-at-large. These efforts have produced an overwhelming sense of employee pride. Ninety-eight percent of our employees reported in the employee feedback survey that they are proud to be a part of our organization.

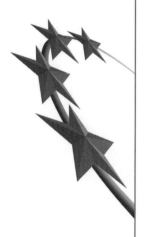

Bristol Hospital

Bristol, Conn.

Mystery shoppers are used by retail stores, airlines, hotels, and restaurants to learn how employees deliver service. Few hospitals have used this method of research for the obvious reason that health care services are difficult for shoppers to access and consume. But Denver Health has overcome this challenge and regularly uses mystery shoppers to offer their perceptions of care and service. Executives and managers use this feedback to praise or correct staff performance, validate assumptions, identify cross-departmental issues, and provide new ideas for service development.

Customer satisfaction can be measured using a variety of methods, most of which rely primarily upon customer recall. Typically, satisfaction surveys ask patients to respond to inquiries about services received days or weeks earlier, thereby introducing recall bias. Denver Health was interested to learn how service was being delivered in "real time" so we developed a Mystery Shopper program.

Denver Health's organizational development (OD) department is responsible for the Mystery Shopper program. We recruit and train shoppers, develop shopper scenarios, distribute shopper reports to managers, and issue a monthly report to our mid-level managers and executive staff.

Shoppers are trained to telephone hospital departments or clinics and interact with hospital staff. Some examples of common scenarios for telephone mystery shoppers include making appointments, getting directions, inquiring about where to park, or confirming the time of an appointment. Sometimes they present challenging problems to the staff so they can evaluate employees' problem-solving or complaint-handling skills. The scenarios used by the shoppers are developed by the manager of OD, often with input from the department managers who can accurately describe likely situations that employees could encounter at the clinics or hospital.

While on-site, shoppers are trained to look for clues to quality, such as the time it took for staff to acknowledge their presence or whether information about safety precautions was volunteered. They note wait times in reception areas and exam rooms and what they observe about staff interactions with other customers and each other.

After their interactions, the shoppers evaluate staff performance and other satisfiers such as the availability of convenient parking and the comfort of waiting areas. Shoppers submit reports of their experiences and meet with the coordinator to share their findings and perceptions.

Managers receive shopper reports within 24 hours and they respond to information contained in the report by commending or coaching staff, validating system issues, or taking corrective actions to remedy service

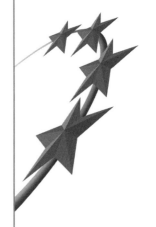

Denver Health

Denver, Colo.

breakdowns. On a form that is returned to the OD department, managers identify their responses to the shopper report.

Often, shoppers are dispatched to shop services that are known to be problematic, based on customer satisfaction surveys, patient representative reports or as identified by managers and executive staff. Directors can request mystery shopping of their departments or services.

To recruit a stable of reliable shoppers, monetary compensation is provided. Shoppers are recruited from senior groups, local colleges, and through advertisements in local newspapers. Students in Denver Health's Clerical Academy serve as mystery shoppers. Their participation enhances their own awareness and understanding of customer service because they are able to experience service from a customer's perspective.

The Mystery Shopper program at Denver Health is one way we measure perceptions of care and service. Included in our measurement efforts are patient focus groups. We convene these groups and interview patients to gain valuable insights that are helpful in guiding our service improvement efforts. We also use a standardized, nationally validated survey to measure patient satisfaction of care received at Denver Health Medical Center and the ambulatory clinics. The results are used to provide a comprehensive picture of satisfaction, identify areas of concern, target improvements, and set employee bonus distributions. Improvement expectations are set by the board and we have a comprehensive customer service plan that addresses staff development, leadership training, rewards and recognition, accountability and complaint management. Patient satisfaction continues to rise and Denver Health's customer service program has been cited locally as a model for other health care organizations.

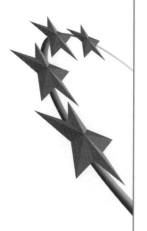

Denver Health

Denver, Colo.

Some departments deliver services that benefit patients or other external customers, but which are delivered directly to internal customers, such as nurses or physicians. Memorial Hospital & Health System of South Bend created a computerized survey to measure internal service satisfaction. Employees can rate the performance of 37 departments and offer their comments or suggestions by accessing the survey through an internal Web site. Since introducing the online survey, the number of users has increased 50% and more than 25 departments have asked to be included in the evaluation.

M emorial Hospital & Health System of South Bend launched a World Class Organization initiative several years ago. Eight teams were created to carry the initiative forward. The Measurement Team targeted ways to measure and report our progress. One of our initiatives was a weekly survey asking nursing unit managers to rate the services delivered by ten key support areas, such as sterile processing and laundry services. This paper-and-pencil survey was unpopular and there was a low compliance rate. In addition, entering data and reporting results were time-consuming. To solve these problems, the Measurement Team created an online instrument to make it easier to access and use, as well as to tabulate the results.

The team spent a year developing the computer program and refining the survey. Ratings are given for promptness, communication, courtesy and consistency in meeting the needs of the internal customer. We decided to extend the capability for all employees to provide feedback, rather than limiting its use to nurse managers. We developed the following guidelines:

Promote the Features and Benefits. We encourage employees to use the survey tool by placing announcements in the newsletter and sending email reminders. We offer prize drawings to encourage wider participation. We were able to promote and demonstrate the value of the survey recently when we sent a letter to all new hires and asked them to rate their experiences during the screening, interviewing and orientation processes. This feedback was given to our human resources department.

Allow Departments to Opt-In. Any department can be added to the survey. Of the 37 departments currently listed on the survey, all but the original ten asked to be included. Because of the automated nature of the survey, the labor to add departments to the survey or to process feedback from a larger number of respondents is negligible.

Clarify the Limitations. This survey is a tool. It is not intended to be a substitute for communication. Respondents are required to provide brief explanations when they offer low ratings. Space for comments is limited to encourage service providers and internal customers to have face-to-face conversations.

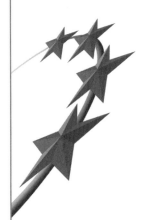

Memorial Hospital of South Bend

South Bend, Ind.

Protect Anonymity and Confidentiality. Total anonymity is not possible because the computer program must be able to verify employment status and prevent people from rating their own department or taking the monthly survey multiple times. But we recognized some people might not give honest feedback if required to leave their name. For each department being rated, the respondent must indicate whether they give permission for the manager to know their identity.

Make Results Accessible. The results of the survey are continuously tabulated and available online. Any employee can see the average rating for any department and the number of respondents for any given month. Only authorized managers and supervisors have access to the comments.

Use Feedback to Recognize Excellence. We knew that if we expected departmental managers and employees to take this survey seriously, we needed to make sure excellence in internal service was recognized and that departments used the feedback. The chief operating officer awards each high-scoring department a banner at the monthly management meeting. High-scoring departments are defined as those with a total average score of 90 or better (the 5-point rating scale is converted to a 100-point reporting scale) with a minimum of five respondents.

The survey has become increasingly valuable to managers and employee participation continues to grow. The average number of people rating each area has increased 50% since its inception. The number of departments participating has almost quadrupled and the average number of awards given out each month has increased 125%. In one recent month, 23 of 37 departments were recognized for high scores.

Memorial Hospital & Health System continues to implement many programs to measure our achievement of World Class Organization status. We consider our internal satisfaction survey process to be a unique method and very effective in encouraging participation and improvement.

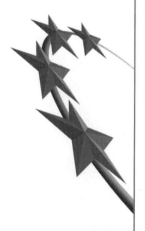

*Memorial
Hospital of
South Bend*

South Bend, Ind.

Receiving the wrong answer to a question is often worse than receiving a discourteous reply or no help at all. The Department of Veterans Affairs New Jersey Health Care System created a centralized information database to improve the accuracy of information offered by employees while interacting with customers. As a result, complaints about triage of information decreased by 62%.

An enabling goal of the Veteran's Administration Strategic Plan is to create an environment that fosters the delivery of One-VA World-Class Service to veterans and their families through effective communication and management of people and technology. But aggregate data obtained from the Consumer Satisfaction sub-council showed that, in the opinion of employees and patients, this goal was not being met at the Department of Veterans Affairs New Jersey Health Care System (VANJHCS). The inability of employees to answer questions about our organization or to direct patients to the correct location within VANJHCS was a big source of patient dissatisfaction. Survey feedback from employees validated their frustrations caused by not having a centralized information database to reference.

The Customer Service Knowledge (CSK) project was implemented to increase patient satisfaction and decrease complaints about employee inability to triage information. Objectives of the project included: 1) providing resources to internal customers (staff and volunteers) so they could deliver exceptional service to external customers, and 2) rewarding employees who demonstrated superior knowledge about the VANJHCS. A CSK Committee comprised of an interdisciplinary team of employees and one volunteer was formed to identify ways to improve access to information about VANJHCS so accurate responses to customers' inquiries could be provided.

With input from employees, patients, union partners, and stakeholders, we identified the need to assemble and organize information about our organization and provide it in written and digital formats. We developed a CSK handbook that is easy to reference and provides accurate triage of information. A distinguishing feature of the handbook involves the use of keywords. A "keyword" is a term that is frequently used by veterans to access services. For example, a veteran might not articulate a service using the internal name, such as PREP, an acronym for Pulmonary Rehabilitation and Empowerment Program. Our research revealed that veterans use no less than 10 different keywords to access PREP, such as breathing, coughing, ventilators, pulmonary, respirators, lung, bronchitis, asthma, emphysema, or oxygen service. CSK Committee members contacted all areas of VANJHCS to determine keywords frequently used by veterans. Keywords now enable staff to relate to our services from the veteran's perspective.

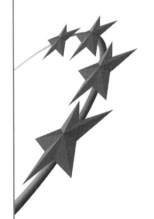

Veterans Affairs
New Jersey
Health Care System

East Orange, N.J.

Handbook sections include a message from the chief executive officer, the mission statement, address, telephone and toll-free directories, public transportation and campus maps, a key word index, information about scheduling appointments and answers to frequently asked questions.

After the handbook was published, classes were offered to teach employees how to use the handbook and the computer application. CSK Committee members wanted to recognize and reward employees who took the initiative to use these new resources. We designed a test, using 25 scenarios and problem-solving activities. Test questions were developed from the database and validated with the assistance of the office of performance management and improvement. A total of 150 employees volunteered to take the test during the pilot phase and first quarter it was offered. Those who pass the test receive a time-off award based on their test scores. A score of 85% to 100% rewards the employee with eight hours time-off; a 70% to 85% score earns four hours time-off. Employees who pass the test also are recognized at an award ceremony and presented with certificates. Two different versions of the test have been standardized and are administered on a quarterly basis.

These resources have contributed to employees' confidence when responding to customers. Complaints about triage of information have decreased by 62% and the number of employees who ask to take the test continues to increase.

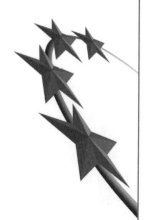

Veterans Affairs
New Jersey
Health Care System

East Orange, N.J.

The willingness of Geisinger Health System to extend accountability for contribution to patient satisfaction to physicians is a demonstration of leadership and commitment. Geisinger trains physicians in clinician-patient communications, monitors performance, and uses patient satisfaction as a compensation criterion. Overall, physicians' scores throughout the system's clinic locations have improved by at least 40 percentile points since the initiative was introduced.

Geisinger Health System believes that service quality is a fundamental performance indicator that everyone affiliated with the system should be constantly working to improve. Senior management considered patient dissatisfaction to be unacceptable for an organization that took pride in hiring "the best" physicians and staff.

A two-person team consisting of a senior physician leader and an administrator leads the Geisinger initiative for physician development. The plan to improve patient satisfaction with Geisinger physicians had components designed to:

- work through both physician and non-physician leadership at all levels, from the chief executive officer to work unit leaders, to make "service excellence to the patient" a priority and part of the physician culture;

- teach specific clinician-patient communication skills to physicians on an ongoing basis using 16 of our own physician champions as faculty;

- measure patient satisfaction on an ongoing basis and provide individual scores and feedback to each physician.

Geisinger sent 16 physicians to The Bayer Institute for Health Care Communication to be trained as faculty capable of teaching communication workshops. The workshops then were offered monthly to all Geisinger physicians and taught by the faculty.

Leadership mandated that all physicians and mid-level providers attend the six-hour workshop titled "Clinician–Patient Communication," and 600 physicians completed this requirement.

The second expectation was that physicians attend a workshop called "Difficult Clinician–Patient Relationships." This requirement is close to being completed, with almost 400 providers attending to date.

A third program, "Connected–Communicating and Computing in the Exam Room," is required for physicians who practice in areas that have an automated outpatient medical record. This workshop is conducted for doctors and nurses and more than 250 have completed the course.

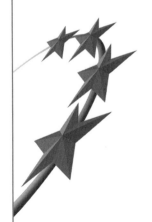

*Geisinger
Health System*
Danville, Pa.

Some 20 physicians who were struggling with communication issues attended a week-long intensive communication training course. Each physician is coached by one of the physician coaches Geisinger selected and trained for the role. In addition, a program has been developed internally to provide ongoing teaching, coaching, and follow-up for all physicians who consistently receive low patient satisfaction scores. We call this program "Common Ground," and it consists of a series of short communication workshops, followed by six months of individual coaching. The workshops contain mini-lectures and observations of clinician-patient interactions on video. The physicians are then videotaped while interacting with patients during role plays. We have made arrangements with a local theater company to supply actors and actresses who role play with physicians for these videotaped exercises.

Sustaining and continuously improving physician performance for high patient satisfaction will only happen if we maintain a strong commitment to service excellence as a cultural attribute. To strengthen this culture, Geisinger leaders have committed to:

- provide all physicians with their own individual patient satisfaction scores, ranked in the largest comparative database obtainable, on an ongoing basis;

- make physician "service excellence" an ongoing leadership initiative;

- offer educational programs that will help physicians further improve their skills and relationships with patients.

Goals are established and success is celebrated. Individual physician patient satisfaction scores are used when evaluating physician performance, and factored into physician compensation. Linking patient satisfaction to individual compensation has been controversial at times but it certainly has sent a strong message to everyone that patient satisfaction is highly valued at Geisinger.

Patient satisfaction scores show the 200 providers on the Danville campus are at the 81st percentile; the 40 providers on the Wilkes-Barre campus are at the 82nd percentile; and 250 "community practice providers" are at the 62nd percentile. This is much improved over the scores two years earlier and all three rankings improved by at least 40 points.

Geisinger's national ranking of physician productivity has improved along with patient satisfaction scores. By plotting all of our doctors on a scatter diagram, we can quantitatively show the correlation between service and productivity. The most populated quadrant of this diagram by far is the one indicating high scores for both.

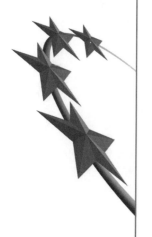

Geisinger Health System

Danville, Pa.

Key words are specific words or phrases used to assure, inform, or impress patients and other customers. Key actions are instructive guidelines for performing specific procedures or conducting routine interactions. Sharp Grossmont Hospital created a multidisciplinary Key Word Action Team to develop key actions and words for employees to use during patient care interactions. Key words and actions have contributed to patient satisfaction and employee confidence.

The Key Word Task Force at Sharp Grossmont Hospital spent a month developing key actions and words for nursing assistants. Nursing assistants were chosen to be among the first to be trained because of their important roles in patient care. Each nursing assistant received a set of laminated cards while attending a class that explained the initiative. The right and wrong ways to use key actions and words were demonstrated by "Key Word People" who performed skits during the class. A videotape of the skits was produced to use in future educational sessions. When the initial rollout to two nursing units was completed, remaining units participated in the program over a period of three months. Subsequently, the task force also developed key words and actions for other departments.

Examples of key words used by nursing assistants are:

- "We will be closing your curtain/door at times to provide for your privacy."

- "For your convenience, here is your call light; if you need anything, please press this button."

- "Someone will be checking on you at least once an hour. Do you have any questions? Is there anything else I can do for you before I leave?"

- "Here is a warm blanket for your comfort."

Examples of key actions used by nursing assistants are:

- Write the nurse's name, your name and the admitting physician's name on the white board before the patient arrives. Also write *"Welcome Mr./Mrs./Ms. _____."*

- Before entering a room, stop, knock, wait for acknowledgment, enter the room, smile and introduce yourself by name and title.

- Give the patient a warm washcloth and dry towel to freshen up before a meal.

- On exiting a patient's room, ensure that the bedside table, telephone, water pitcher, and call light are within the patient's reach.

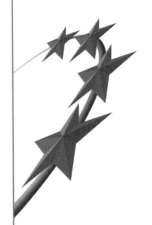

Sharp Grossmont Hospital

La Mesa, Calif.

The task force developed "Key Word Kash" as a way to recognize employees when they use key actions and words. The "kash"—small cards that read, *"I'm the key to patient/customer satisfaction!"*—can be collected and redeemed for a variety of rewards.

Key words and actions enhance perceptions of our professionalism and responsiveness. This initiative contributed to scores for inpatient satisfaction progressively improving from the 27th percentile to the 62nd percentile on one unit.

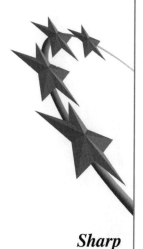

Sharp Grossmont Hospital

La Mesa, Calif.

In an article published by the *Arizona Republic* about nursing shortages in the Phoenix metropolitan area, Banner Thunderbird Medical Center was described as "Pleasantville." Banner Thunderbird employs lots of pleasant people but this distinction was earned by persistence and hard work. Wanting to build a culture where it is fun to work, leaders realized they needed to "reinvent" themselves and become more participative and communicative. One of the programs they used to inform, educate, and engage employees is known as "60 Minutes."

Life has not always been so pleasant at Banner Thunderbird Medical Center. Five years ago, a threat of unionization was growing and the staff was not engaged. Members of our leadership team embarked on a campaign to reinvent themselves. They were perceived to be "lean and mean" administrators. They wanted to be known as participative leaders dedicated to creating a culture characterized by open communication, fun, spirit, and celebration.

The culture was reformed around these goals. Leaders make rounds daily. Departments are encouraged to recognize staff with monetary rewards and celebrations. We regularly host parties and events, sometimes featuring entertainment provided by the Thunderbird Band. When this group was formed, our CEO at the time played the keyboard.

One of the most notable contributions to this turnaround has been a one hour production known as "60 Minutes." Based on the CBS television program *"60 Minutes,"* the show is anchored by our CEO, and we have taken a few liberties with the content and format to make the show informative and entertaining.

The format is structured to educate viewers about five strategies: 1) relationships, 2) growth, 3) finance, 4) patient safety/clinical excellence, and 5) service excellence. Some of this information can be considered dry until the audience is shown videotaped role plays. For example, one of the segments educated staff on where smoking was permitted on campus. Patient complaints about having to walk through clouds of cigarette smoke when entering or exiting the hospital gave us the story concept.

A twisted tale called *"The Smoking Zone"* based on the *"Twilight Zone"* television series was narrated by our director of planning. In a deep and resonant voice with a British accent, "Rog Hurling" told the tale of a visitor who just wanted to smoke. The visitor, a dry and cracked "Mr. Bill" clay figure that was able to blow smoke from his mouth, was caught smoking in all the wrong places. Staff was shown telling Mr. Bill where he was allowed to smoke. The intent of this video was to let the staff know that it is appropriate to inform visitors and employees about our smoking policy and to guide them to approved areas.

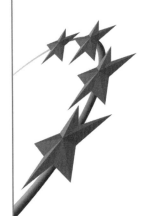

Banner Thunderbird Medical Center

Glendale, Ariz.

There are at least five fun videos in each quarterly show. We've produced music videos for recruiting and service excellence and financial weather reports. One of our materials management skits featured French-Canadian hockey players. To discover new talent, casting calls are made to the staff of the hospital and auditions are held.

These shows are perhaps the most important communication tool the hospital uses to reach its employees. Nearly 1,800 of 2,200 total employees voluntarily attend these shows, which are held at various times to make it accessible to all shifts. At the end of each show, prizes are given and the host takes questions from the audience. Attendees are asked to complete a survey at the conclusion of the program.

These presentations are repeated 30 to 40 times each quarter, which indicates the level of commitment we extend to communication and interaction at Banner Thunderbird. Through this program, the hospital has been able to reinforce its core messages and add to the culture of honest and open communication.

Communication is one of the qualities of our culture that has helped to build employee confidence and commitment. Banner Thunderbird has the lowest staff turnover in the Phoenix market. We are the fastest growing hospital in Arizona, and employees have become our greatest asset in recruiting new staff to "Pleasantville."

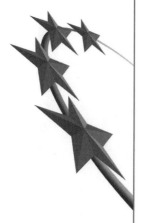

Banner
Thunderbird
Medical Center

Glendale, Ariz.

Baptist Health Care developed a unique method of communication designed to reinforce continuous learning. This discipline calls for 10 minutes to be set aside five days a week to allow department managers to introduce scripted lessons covering a wide range of topics and known as the "BHC Daily." The depth of Baptist Health Care's commitment to keep employees engaged in "what's happening" and "what's important" is demonstrated by the fact that more than 40 hours are devoted to organizational communications every year.

Baptist Health Care (BHC) introduced the BHC Daily to help us sustain a culture of service and operational excellence. The idea was conceived after we visited Ritz-Carlton Hotels to benchmark our performance in organizational communications and leadership development. Ritz-Carlton uses daily "line-ups" to instruct employees and reinforce service principles and organizational values. We adapted this concept as a "continuous learning tool" that enables BHC to increase organizational knowledge and service performance in a cost-effective and time-efficient manner.

At the end of each week, all department managers receive an electronic file containing the following week's daily scripts. Each department or business unit sets a specific time to gather and share the BHC Daily. This time is known as the "line-up" where employees literally stand for the 10-minute learning session.

Line-ups take place every day throughout the organization at varying times. Employees are encouraged to join in if they are visiting another department at line-up time. Each script provides information on the topic for the day, discussion questions to encourage interaction among the team members or to solicit employee feedback, and an inspirational quote. Sometimes we brief employees on national health care news, share customer comments or recognize departments and individuals. Other times we reinforce our mission, vision, values, service principles, or standards of performance.

Department managers are encouraged to make the line-up fun and often include activities like doing the "hokey-pokey" or sponsoring a homemade hat-making contest. It is also a time when department managers can publicly recognize employees who have performed exceptional service.

The BHC Daily issues special bulletins when situations warrant prompt dissemination of "breaking news." One issue of the BHC Daily shared comforting words from the governor of Florida and our chief executive officer regarding the terrorist attacks. Another issue was devoted to soliciting feedback from participants.

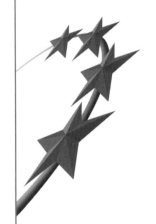

Baptist Health Care

Pensacola, Fla.

The following quotes are in response to the question, *"What is your favorite component of the BHC Daily and why?"*

- "I like the interaction it generates. There are four small departments in our suite that participate together. We have certainly bonded due to the program."

- "It has brought our department closer as a family or unit–and also communication between employee-employee and management-employee is lots better."

- "Quote for the day–leaves us with something to think about. They are well-chosen and varied."

The BHC Daily is a team effort; an advisory committee meets monthly to outline the topics for the coming month. Each member of the committee solicits feedback from throughout the organization, such as employee stories and examples of service excellence that can be included in the BHC Daily.

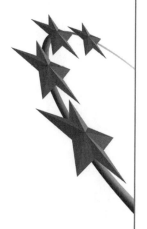

Baptist Health Care

Pensacola, Fla.

From immediate "on the spot" recognition to programs focused on rewarding exceptional acts that reflect organizational values, there are many ways to reinforce behaviors that contribute to satisfying customers. Hackensack University Medical Center uses a "5 Star Care" recognition program to liberally recognize employees. Close to 10,000 citations for 5 Star Care were distributed during the first year of this program.

A group of employees and managers convened to develop a plan that would heighten staff's awareness of Hackensack University Medical Center commitment to exceed patient expectations and recognize employees for their contributions in achieving that outcome. The most sensible approach was to incorporate our patient satisfaction survey process with an employee recognition program. The 5 Star Care campaign was launched with the following objectives, to:

- educate patients regarding the survey process and communicate to each patient the level of care they can expect;

- inform management when patient expectations are not met;

- provide education to hospital staff regarding the satisfaction survey process;

- continue to ensure a patient-focused culture by rewarding and recognizing employees who exemplify our standards of care;

- improve employee satisfaction and morale by continuously celebrating and acknowledging positive behaviors;

- focus management's attention on reinforcing our standards of care.

A series of bulletin board presentations about the 5 Star Care program was prepared and sent to all departments to be displayed in view of patients, visitors, and staff. A welcome card was created. This card is given to patients by the nurse manager and it expresses our best wishes, explains the medical center intent to provide excellent care and service, and instructs the patient how to let us know if their expectations are not met.

Patients are sent satisfaction surveys seven days after discharge. The survey asks patients to rate their level of satisfaction with the services they received. Patients often recognize employees by name and offer examples of exemplary care on these surveys. In addition, patients frequently mail greeting cards to units or to employees thanking them for their care. Patients also communicate compliments through phone calls and letters to administration. These channels provide ways to collect the identities of individuals who are then recognized with one or more of following citations:

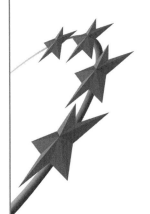

Hackensack University Medical Center

Hackensack, N.J.

5 Star Care Certificates. The consumer affairs department issues 5 Star Care certificates to employees who receive compliments through any form of communication from patients or family members (i.e., mail, survey and phone). Managers are notified of this recognition.

5 Star Care Coupons. When managers want to acknowledge behaviors that exemplify our quality standards, they can issue 5 Star Care coupons. These coupons are worth points and can be redeemed for beverages, meals, manicures, massages, etc.).

Five Star Care Pins. Gold star pins are presented at monthly management meetings to employees receiving five or more certificates and/or coupons during a three month period. Once employees receive five pins, they become the medical center's Employees of the Month.

Most Valuable Team Member Awards. Every month, three employees are recognized as Most Valuable Team Members; annually, one employee is chosen as Most Valuable Team Member of the Year.

We believe employee recognition has contributed to employee satisfaction, recruitment and morale. In a comparative database, HUMC was ranked on these following dimensions:

- My level of pride in HUMC – 97th percentile

- How I would rate HUMC as an employer – 97th percentile

- Likelihood of encouraging my friends to apply – 96th percentile

- My attitude about working at HUMC – 96th percentile

The 5 Star Care program contributes to HUMC's ability to acknowledge those who provide outstanding service to our patients and customers. Close to 10,000 recognition awards were issued to deserving employees in the first ycar of the program.

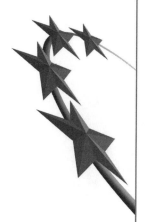

**Hackensack
University
Medical Center**

Hackensack, N.J.

The concept behind Bayhealth Medical Center's "You've Been Caught" program is catching and rewarding staff for responding to the needs of others. A toolkit was developed to make it easy for directors to reward employees after catching them in the act of sustaining the medical center's patient-centered care philosophy and contributing to teamwork.

The Customer Service Liaison Team at Bayhealth Medical Center meets monthly to discuss customer service practices, policies, issues, and challenges. We wanted to implement a recognition program that would reward employees, on the spot, for contributing to exceptional customer service. We developed the procedures for the "You've Been Caught" program and designed a toolkit that looks like a miniature doctor's bag. Over 200 toolkits—filled with items such as movie tickets and gift certificates to Bath and Body Works, Dunkin' Donuts, Dairy Queen, the local car wash, golf driving range, batting cage, and bowling alley—were distributed to directors and managers. The bags also contained candy bars, mints, and granola bars. The recipients were given one specific task: *"Go out and reward staff for doing the right things."*

To sustain the program, we look for new gifts to distribute and ways to keep the program strong. Each person who receives a gift is eligible for a $50 gift certificate that can be redeemed at a local shopping mall. This certificate is awarded at a monthly drawing.

During the past 18 months, we have distributed over 1,500 gifts to employees who have been caught. When we began, we had an approved budget of $2,000 to spend. Within months, we realized the program was catching on and increased the budget to $10,000.

Recognizing staff promotes teamwork and reinforces customer service. Employees who are caught receive a gift and their name is mentioned in our quarterly newsletter. Employees enjoy the gifts and they appreciate being noticed. The attention seems to provide as much value as the gift itself.

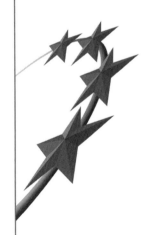

Bayhealth
Medical Center

Dover, Del.

Learning & Leadership
Oak Leaf Awards Honor Heroes

A symbol that personifies ideals and attributes a deeper significance to an award enhances the perceived value. Oak leaves symbolize strength, military glory, immortality, and insignia of rank for all branches of the United States armed forces. Veterans Administration New Jersey Health Care System created the Oak Leaf Awards program to reward employees who deliver exceptional service and demonstrate the organization's values. The Oak Leaf Award is symbolic of the exceptional service that has been given to the country by veterans.

A customer service plan was developed by the Veterans Administration New Jersey Health Care System's (VANJHCS's) office of public affairs to achieve a service culture that reflects our values and symbolizes the veteran experience. We received survey results on an annual basis and realized that more frequent patient feedback was needed. Another shortfall related to employee dissatisfaction with rewards and recognition.

The Oak Leaf Awards program provides more frequent customer feedback on service quality delivered by providers and staff. The program also satisfies the need to offer positive feedback to employees whose performance exceeds customer expectations.

Oak Leaf Awards are given to employees who have been cited in written correspondence such as letters or Oak Leaf Award nomination forms. Any veteran, guest, or employee can submit a nomination. The Oak Leaf Awards program consists of four levels: Pewter Oak Leaf, Bronze Oak Leaf, Silver Oak Leaf, and Gold Oak Leaf. The frequency of citation determines award level attainment. Recipients of the award receive pewter, bronze, silver, or gold pins and can make selections of gifts from award catalogues. Time off is awarded at the gold level.

We have shared the Oak Leaf Awards program with the veteran community through the Stakeholders Advisory Group. Stakeholders are veterans who have served in leadership positions or veteran advocacy groups. Promotional materials have been distributed internally and externally. Two volunteers telephone customers to verify information and express our appreciation for the nominations.

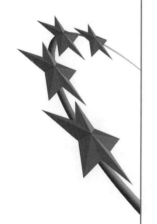

Veterans Affairs New Jersey Health Care System

East Orange, N.J.

A search on Amazon.com using the keyword "leadership" produces more than 100,000 book titles. Obviously, there is no shortage of leadership advice, but few hospitals and health systems invest in solid, competency-based programs to build leadership performance. At Guthrie Health, leadership development is a business strategy. Leaders earn certification by participating in courses and completing other related requirements that help to assure leadership performance is aligned with the strategic direction of the enterprise.

Quality patient care and customer satisfaction remain the fundamental goals by which Guthrie measures its success. Leaders work together to improve the patient experience, expand market share, improve financial performance, and strengthen employee morale. To meet these challenges, leaders need to develop expanded capabilities. Through a series of focus groups, conversations with leaders, and benchmark comparisons of best practices, we identified 11 leadership competencies that would most directly enable us to achieve our strategic goals.

Once the competencies were defined, we developed a tool that measures performance in each of these areas. After completing this segment of the evaluation process, leaders and their leadership partners developed professional development plans that were targeted to close performance gaps.

An advisory board, consisting of senior leaders from Guthrie Health and Guthrie Clinic, helped to identify the requirements of leadership development and performance. Guthrie leaders are expected to participate in a certification process that includes: 1) four required core courses, 2) four strategic alignment courses, and 3) a minimum of 12 elective courses linked to strengthening core leadership competencies.

The elective courses are categorized under three learning tracks relating to: 1) delivering results, 2) working with people, and 3) developing personal effectiveness. In addition to the core courses and electives, time-sensitive learning solutions supporting the execution of specific business fundamentals or resulting from shifts in strategic direction are scheduled as needed.

In addition to classroom learning, leaders can meet elective requirements by participating in online learning, satellite conferences, and external education programs. Multiple resources supporting professional development are also available from our in-house library and include books, professional journals, audio tapes, videotapes, CD-ROMs, etc. We have also identified web sites on the subject of leadership.

Newly appointed leaders attend a one-day orientation program that covers Guthrie's values-centered culture, performance improvement process, patient/employee satisfaction goals, financial principles, organizational

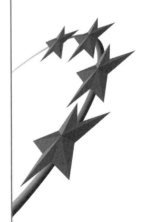

Guthrie Health

Sayre, Pa.

resources, emotional intelligence traits, leadership philosophy, and leadership development. This course is offered quarterly and is taught by senior leaders.

To support leadership development, we have developed reinforcement systems and tools including:

Performance Evaluation. Annual performance evaluations are completed, performance gaps are identified, and development plans are updated to ensure continuous improvement in leadership performance measured against the 11 competency areas.

Performance Feedback. Guthrie leaders are encouraged to participate in a 360-degree feedback process. The results of that assessment are incorporated into the development plan and are also used to chart progress over time.

Assessment Tools. Emotional Quotient Maps and DISC® profiles are tools that give leaders the opportunity to self-assess traits of emotional intelligence and behavioral style. Elective courses that specifically address these traits are offered.

Participant Evaluation. Level 1, 2, and 3 evaluations are used to improve class content, revise and update materials, and assess needs.

Other Incentives. Leaders can take advantage of tuition and other financial reimbursements once they complete coursework at local colleges or universities, attend professional conferences and workshops, and present best practices at conferences.

The organization benefits from strong leadership and the most direct beneficiaries are employees. We continue to link employee satisfaction, workforce commitment, and organizational performance indicators to the contributing competencies from our leadership model to measure the impact of leadership development.

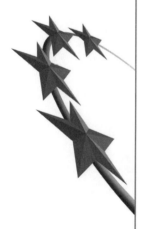

**Guthrie
Health**

Sayre, Pa.

Staffing shortages have focused attention on employee recruitment and retention but health care organizations cannot hope to remain viable unless similar attention is given to succession planning and leadership development. The University of Kentucky Hospital recognized the need to begin preparing up-and-coming leaders so its capability to recruit and retain committed staff in the future remains strong.

The Leadership Mentoring program at the University of Kentucky Hospital (UK) is designed to unite a willing experienced leader with a willing junior leader who wishes to gain vision and learn from the senior leader's experiences. The objectives of the program are to support the hospital in attracting, developing, and retaining highly competent and skilled staff, and to:

- reduce the turnover rate of leadership positions;

- prepare leaders to fill the vacant positions of leaders resigning or retiring;

- reduce the learning curve and improve productivity of new leaders;

- foster a climate of learning and trust among leaders.

Four leaders were selected to become mentors after a rigorous application and selection process. Mentor candidates were required to meet the selection criteria that we established at the outset of the program. They were interviewed by senior administrative officers of the hospital, medical center, and university. These four designees represented three levels of the management hierarchy; administrators, directors, and managers. Following this selection, the application process was opened to candidates seeking to become apprentice leaders. Four were selected; one director and three staff members. The mentors and apprentices were paired after the apprentice leaders each ranked their individual preferences for mentors. The only requirement was that mentors and apprentices could not be from the same service area.

The mentor relationships began in September and ended in August. Mentor and apprentice leaders were expected to meet once a month. The apprentice leader was required to submit quarterly progress reports, and both parties in the relationship completed evaluations of the process at the end of the year.

An orientation program and mentoring guide were developed to help structure the relationships, goals, and objectives. A midyear luncheon was held, at which time the participants reviewed their progress and offered suggestions to the program leaders. At the end of the year, another luncheon was held to review and celebrate successes. Top ratings were given by all

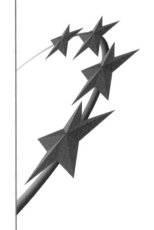

University of Kentucky Hospital
Lexington, Ky.

mentors and apprentice leaders based on their evaluations of the value of the program, the benefit to the organization, their satisfaction with their partner, and their personal development.

Three of the four apprentice leaders have already been promoted to leadership positions within the organization. The fourth apprentice was already in a significant leadership position when she applied for the program, but wanted to learn better communication skills from her mentor.

Two service directors agreed to become new mentors and the four mentors signed on for another year. Six new apprentice leaders were accepted into the program. Our structured program continues to evolve but it has already paid dividends by preparing leaders to assume larger roles in the future.

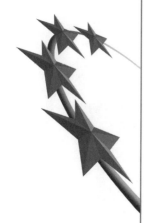

University of Kentucky Hospital

Lexington, Ky.

As San Diego's largest home care agency, Sharp Home Care serves a diverse patient population and employs a culturally diverse team of employees. A month-long event consisting of programs and activities was sponsored to build knowledge and respect for the cultural differences of both customers and staff. Celebrate and Rejoice in Diversity has had a positive impact, not only within this unit of Sharp HealthCare, but throughout the system. One hundred percent of those who participated confirmed that they learned something that will influence how they interact with patients or co-workers in the future.

Our dedicated, caring employees are united in our mission and motivated by our vision to make Sharp Home Care the best place to work, the best place to receive health care, and the best place to practice medicine. Celebrate and Rejoice in Diversity is an extension of our commitment to foster understanding and respect within and outside of our workplace and to value our differences. This, in turn, broadens our potential to develop fulfilling relationships with the patients we serve and our colleagues.

Celebrate and Rejoice in Diversity was a month-long experience, made up of programs, presentations, and activities planned and executed by a team of 12 representatives from different areas within our agency.

During the initial stages of planning our Celebrate and Rejoice in Diversity program, we discovered that a large percentage of our 258 employees are bi-lingual; no less than 18 different languages are spoken by our staff. With such a diverse staff, we were afforded the opportunity to easily interview them, and we learned many interesting perspectives related to attitudes and beliefs about illness, the roles family members assume as caregivers, and rituals and beliefs about healing. We posted these answers so everyone could benefit from the insights they shared. The interview questions included:

- What is your culture's attitude toward illness?

- How do you feel about health care providers who are not of the same cultural background or gender?

- How do you or your family perceive the role of the home care provider and what are your expectations of them?

- What is an example of a behavior that would be a cultural faux pas?

- How does the family or extended family play a part in planning or administering health care treatments?

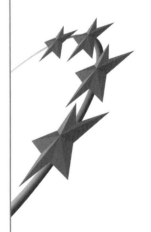

*Sharp
Home Care*

San Diego, Calif.

We launched Celebrate and Rejoice in Diversity by providing the staff with materials and instruction to create a Mini~Me. We asked them to select a country of association, either by ancestry or special interest. To create the Mini~Me, staff members chose one of 12 paper dolls; each had a different skin tone. They then placed a photograph of their face on the head and decorated the body with articles associated with their country of choice, as well as with items unique to their personalities such as hobbies, roles, pets, children, and interests. These were displayed at the final Celebrate and Rejoice in Diversity event at the end of the month. In anticipation of that event, we gave staff a blank recipe card that read:

Don your aprons. Shine your pans.
Whip up an ethnic dish with your magic hands.
Share the recipe from your country of choice
so everyone can have a taste and rejoice.
April 30th is the date.
We'll munch and crunch, so don't be late!

The finale of Celebrate and Rejoice in Diversity included a poster session. We displayed 35 different posters and distributed written handouts. A map of San Diego County and its cultural clusters was titled, "Sharp Home Care Serving a Diverse Population." Nine posters related information about the patient populations we most frequently serve. Posters and handouts also provided information regarding communication styles; family; social and work relationships; health values and beliefs; health customs and practices; history of holidays and holy days; dietary practices; pregnancy and childbirth; death and dying; and family traditions.

In addition to the poster session, a Power Point® presentation, "Defining and Refining Cultural Sensitivity and Competency in Health Care," was also scheduled. This focused on cultural sensitivity and competency, tolerance, challenges for providing culturally competent health care and solutions to improve care. A second phase of the program titled "Clear Communication and Cultural Awareness in Health Care" was also offered. Staff who attended the poster session and the presentations earned one continuing education unit. Participants received a diversity lapel pin to place on their nametags to represent their participation in Celebrate and Rejoice in Diversity.

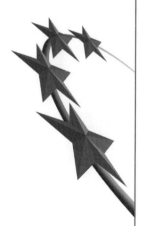

Sharp Home Care

San Diego, Calif.

Concurrent with these events, the "Taste of Diversity International Potluck" supper took place. Staff brought ethnic dishes and recipes to share. The room was decorated with the Mini~Me's, flags of the world, and dolls from different countries. Music from around the world played in the background. World and U.S. maps were displayed side by side. Staff wrote their names on red and white flag pins. They placed the red flags on their country of ancestry and the white flags on their hometown. At the conclusion of the potluck, recipe cards were compiled into a cookbook and distributed to employees.

Our medical campus encompasses four major hospitals, as well as numerous clinics and medical groups stretching across the county, and employs 17,000 people. The opportunity to share Celebrate and Rejoice in Diversity with other entities of Sharp HealthCare has served to increase awareness and positive interactions. The focus of our presentations is altered with consideration for a specific department's scope of practice. For example, the presentation at the mental health facility focused more on health care practices and cultural beliefs regarding mental illness, while the presentation for hospice focused on cultural practices related to death and dying.

We assembled a quick reference guide on diversity and copies have been widely distributed. When confronted by confusing situations, staff can reference this spiral-bound resource for suggestions on how to respond.

In home care, every patient we encounter is asked, "Is there anything I need to know about your spiritual beliefs that would impact the service we provide or your ability to fully participate in your treatment?" We continue to become more culturally sensitive by listening to our customers and responding to their needs and expectations.

Our next phase of diversity training will focus on religious practices including history, dietary restrictions, holy days, birthing practices, death rituals, celebrations, holidays, the power of prayer, healers, and alternative medicine within culturally diverse populations. We are currently putting together a diversity toolkit for distribution when this program is launched.

Celebrate and Rejoice in Diversity has had a positive impact and raised the awareness of all who have had the opportunity to participate in it. Evaluation surveys revealed that 100% of attendees had learned something new that would change the way they interacted with co-workers and patients.

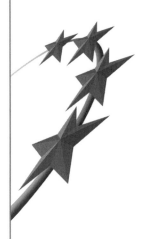

Sharp
Home Care
San Diego, Calif.

American heritage is richly diverse but early generations of immigrants were very adaptive, forsaking language and traditions to assimilate into an evolving but established American culture. As a result, individuals who now live in extended care facilities may not understand the cultural distinctions and practices of employees who work there. Providence Mount St. Vincent created a Diversity Committee to promote awareness and celebrate the hospital's culturally-diverse workforce.

The Diversity Committee was formed at Providence Mount St. Vincent (The Mount) to celebrate the people who serve the community of residents who live at The Mount and their families. The goal of the committee is to bring awareness and education regarding the wonderfully diverse workforce employed at The Mount. Using three points of emphasis—education, food and entertainment—the committee organizes events, publishes educational materials, and combines fun with learning about others and more about ourselves.

The Diversity Committee publishes a newsletter focusing on cultural events. The newsletter features stories and information about various cultures, traditions, and lifestyles from around the world. Past issues have featured the Mexican celebration of Cinco de Mayo; the Chinese New Year; traditional Thanksgiving as celebrated by the North American settlers; Ramadan and the Muslim religion; and the land and customs of Ethiopia. Recipes, employee profiles, history, and local connections to far-off lands are regular features of the newsletter.

Annually around the 4th of July, the Diversity Committee coordinates a Parade of Nations. Staff members wear the clothing of their native lands and carry the flag of their country of origin in a parade around the facility. This ends in a fashion show on our outdoor patio. After the parade and fashion show, employees enjoy a Food Feast featuring foods representative of their native countries prepared by employees to share with all.

Outcomes are difficult to measure quantitatively, but there are evident qualities that can be viewed and experienced daily in the wonderful, caring, inclusive culture at The Mount.

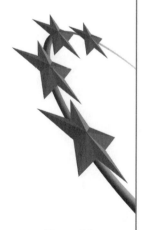

Providence Mount St. Vincent

Seattle, Wash.

Diversity, as both a value and a strategy, requires attentive planning to assure integration into the practices, communications, and competencies of the organization. PinnacleHealth System demonstrates its commitment to diversity in a variety of ways. The system, which serves more than 500,000 patients of varying cultural and ethnic backgrounds, formed a Cultural Diversity Committee to expand its relationships with people of different cultures in the community and within the organization.

The Cultural Diversity Committee at PinnacleHealth System is comprised of employees who represent the diversity of our customers and employees. Four subcommittees were established to address cultural diversity as it relates to: 1) education, training, and competency development, 2) communications, 3) employee relations, and 4) development/funding. This committee has introduced numerous ways cultural awareness and appreciation can be extended.

To proudly represent PinnacleHealth System in the community, our employees attend community events such as The Onganzi Fair and Hispanic Heritage Month celebrations. Recruiters attend job fairs that focus on diverse or minority populations to demonstrate our system's interest in recruiting attendees to join our team. Notices about cultural observances and special events are published in employee and patient education newsletters. A cultural diversity Web site, posting events, calendars, and other facts related to cultural diversity, can be accessed from the system's Intranet.

A Cultural Health Action Team (CHAT) was commissioned to help create an environment in which all of our customers would feel welcome. CHAT strives to promote care that is sensitive and responsive to the varied cultural and spiritual beliefs of our customers. Cultural diversity training has been introduced as segments of leadership training and new employee orientation. Tools and resources such as books, videos, and self-study modules on cultural diversity are readily available to managers. A rotating display of culturally and ethnically diverse artwork by local artists hangs in the main corridor of the hospital. This display has generated an enthusiastic reaction from staff, patients, and visitors who are able to purchase pieces of the collection.

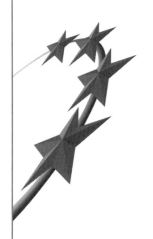

PinnacleHealth

Harrisburg, Pa.

Employee satisfaction = customer satisfaction. A similar tenet, healthy employees = productive employees, is fueling the adoption of wellness programs to benefit the workforce. Wake Forest University Baptist Medical Center created an incentive-based wellness program for its large workforce. Employees receive paid time off to participate in the programs and activities.

Wake Forest University Baptist Medical Center established Action Health to administer an incentive-based employee wellness program that supports and enhances the physical, mental, and spiritual well-being of our employees. The program is available to the more than 11,000 employees of the system's member institutions, including Wake Forest University School of Medicine and North Carolina Baptist Hospitals, Inc.

Our incentive-based plan, called the Health Incentive Program, rewards employees for participating in education, disease prevention, and health enhancement activities. Employees can access educational programs, health assessment, and individual counseling to help them achieve their personal wellness goals. We sponsor educational programs on nutrition, cooking, physical activity, stress management, parenting, and financial planning. Employees receive paid time off to attend health education classes and are eligible to win cash drawings when they receive flu vaccines or complete personal wellness profiles. The staff coordinates weight loss, smoking cessation, blood pressure screening and management, cholesterol monitoring, and exercise programs. Action Health distributes a variety of publications including a monthly wellness newsletter, self-care manuals, and other health-related brochures.

We have received a number of state and national awards for our initiatives to practice what we preach at Wake Forest University Baptist Medical Center. The program has been recognized by the Governor's Council on Physical Fitness and has received several awards for its innovative practices, including the Mother-Friendly Business Award and Well Workplace Awards given by the Wellness Council of America.

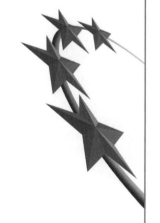

Wake Forest University Baptist Medical Center

Winston – Salem, N.C.

Offering stress management and other holistic and alternative programs to employees can help prevent or heal staff burnout. Hackensack University Medical Center developed "Success Over Stress" to anchor the institution to the values-based philosophy that a hospital can best serve its patients, employees, and community by providing medical care in a nurturing environment.

Taking care of our caregivers is one of the top priorities of Hackensack University Medical Center (HUMC) because it enhances employee morale, promotes a healthier atmosphere for employees and the patients and families they care for, and provides staff with ways to cope with the busy and demanding pace of health care.

HUMC provides a full-day lifestyle stress management program for employees. Offered through the Center for Health and Healing, the Success Over Stress (SOS) program is designed to heal the healers. It integrates modalities such as stress management skills, therapeutic massage, reflexology, holistic nutrition, mind-body medicine, meditation, guided imagery, hypnosis, Tai Chi/Qigong, Svaroopa Yoga, Reiki, and drumming. SOS includes educational and experiential sessions that help to develop a foundation for self-care. The following experiential sessions describe just some of the modalities that are used in the program:

Meditation/Guided Imagery. Staff members learn how to use sitting postures, imagery, and breathing to obtain states of focused or mindful attention. The deep relaxation of meditation helps to quiet the mind and provide a sense of inner balance. Nothing exemplifies the mind-body connection more than visualization imagery. Composed of images in the mind that are made up from one or more of the five senses, the imagination allows one to see, hear, touch, taste, and smell that which is not present in the immediate environment. These images can elicit the same physiologic reactions as if what is imagined is actually present.

Drumming. Simple hand drum rhythms can promote physical, emotional, and spiritual healing. Drumming helps to release anger and create joy, alter brain rhythms, induce meditation and trance, and provide deep and sacred healing. As the participants begin to beat their drums, they naturally align in harmony with each other. The drumming circle is a reminder that we all work together for the purpose of health and healing.

Tai Chi/Qigong. As a Chinese Taoist martial art form of meditation in movement, Tai Chi/Qigong combines mental concentration, coordinated breathing, and a series of slow, graceful body movements.

Hackensack
University
Medical Center

Hackensack, N.J.

Journal Writing. Staff members learn how to use intuition and creativity through journaling. Each staff member is encouraged to purchase a new journal in which to record ideas, words, thoughts, reflections, and unanswered questions.

Humor. The SOS program teaches participants to think optimistically and use humor to experience more joy in their every day lives.

The medical center offers stress management programs that are tailored to specific disciplines, including oncology, geriatrics, pediatrics, and emergency medicine, so staff members can receive help in dealing with particular types of patients or situations.

The program comes to a close with a meditation, at which time participants reflect upon the experiences of the session. This program allows staff immediate stress management modalities within their own work environment to foster self-care. Staff members express gratitude for a humanistic administrative approach to stress management.

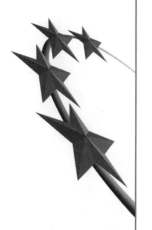

Hackensack University Medical Center

Hackensack, N.J.

As a provider delivering health care in one of the fastest growing communities in the United States, NCH Healthcare System identified that a growing portion of its workforce could not speak English. Many of these employees had the desire to learn but lacked access to instruction. NCH employees willingly volunteered to support their fellow team members and became English language tutors.

According to the 2000 census, Naples, Fla., was the second fastest growing metropolitan area in the United States during the previous decade. As NCH Healthcare System grew to meet the increased demand for services, many good, hard-working individuals who could not speak or read English joined our team. A bid for individuals who were interested in becoming English tutors produced 18 volunteers. Managers and front-line staff came together to provide tutoring support to those who needed help with language.

Assisted by an experienced tutor and linguistics expert, the tutors spent three afternoons practicing language techniques using Laubach instructional methods. Tutors were paired with students and met twice weekly. The sessions were held over lunch and the hospital provided the meal so both students and tutors would miss only one hour of work each week.

Without a doubt, this program has provided an exceptional experience for everyone. Students are visibly more confident and seem to enjoy engaging with others to practice their new skills. Both students and tutors have learned a great deal from each other about their respective heritages. They have bonded and the friendships will endure.

Due to the demand for this program, a second class of tutors has begun. When it concludes, this program will have enriched the lives of more 70 students and tutors.

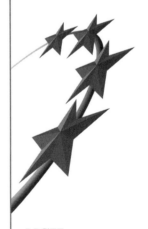

NCH Healthcare System

Naples, Fla.

Although lobbyists and spokespersons for specialty associations do a good job of articulating issues and representing various constituencies to legislators, sometimes it is good to take the initiative to educate politicians and the community. Leaders and nursing staff of Carondelet St. Joseph's Hospital sponsored a program called "Walk-a-Mile With a Nurse" to give community leaders and state legislators the opportunity to learn the facts about the nursing shortage and to experience a nurse's typical workday.

The nation is currently experiencing a critical nursing shortage that is projected to become more acute within the next few years. Arizona is among states experiencing unique challenges with a rapidly aging workforce. Nursing is not seen as an attractive career choice among the youth of today. With the ever-present publicity about this crisis, St. Joseph's Hospital nursing staff planned a program to educate community leaders and legislators.

We conducted a program called "Walk-a-Mile With a Nurse" during Nurse's Week. We invited 11 participants to our facility to hear presentations on the national nursing shortage and how we, and other hospitals, are putting strategies into place to deal with the situation.

Each participant was paired with a nurse from various departments, including critical care, neonatal intensive care, and the emergency department. Following the presentations, our guests were escorted by their nurse partners to the respective departments where they actually worked alongside the nurse for 90 minutes to observe our work and its complexities. At the end of the 90-minute bedside experience with the nurse, participants reassembled for debriefing and evaluation. The dynamics that occurred were astonishing. Many guests expressed a desire to spend more time with the nurses. The dialogue that took place was educational and supportive relationships and bonds were formed. Our state legislators invited their nurse partners to spend a day with them at the state capitol, and commitments were made to stay in touch.

Program evaluations were completed by all guests and nurse partners and all rated the program as excellent. Our nurses were ecstatic about this opportunity to showcase their work. Our greatest success resulted in the procurement of $100,000 from our Foundation to fund nursing scholarships because two of our board members who participated in this program recognized the great need for more nurses.

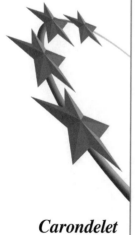

*Carondelet
St. Joseph's
Hospital*

Tucson, Ariz.

CHAPTER 8
RECRUITMENT & RETENTION

RECRUITMENT & RETENTION

Training for health-related careers is offered to at-risk youths by University Medical Center and the Roosevelt–UMC Academy. Roosevelt High School students participate in activities designed to give capable young adults exposure to health careers and employment experience. The high school has a dropout rate of 40%, but one student of 20 dropped out of the first graduating class of this three year program. Of those, 13 went on to complete training to become certified nursing assistants, and four graduates currently work in permanent positions at the medical center.

When it comes to education and future career opportunities, the youth in our community is faced with a number of challenges and barriers. Fresno's unemployment rate is three times higher than that of the state. The percentage of persons under the age of 18 who live in poverty is third highest in the state. California has the third highest rate of juveniles in custody among 50 states. Fresno County is the third most culturally diverse county in the nation. Fresno Unified School District has identified more than 100 languages as the "major source language" in the home and approximately 47,000 "limited English proficient" students are enrolled in Fresno County schools. School dropout rates are higher in Fresno County (4.3%) than California as a whole (2.9%). Perhaps most compelling is the fact that, according to school officials, Roosevelt High School in Fresno has a 40% dropout rate.

In response to these issues, Community Medical Centers, of which University Medical Center (UMC) is a part, formed a unique partnership with Roosevelt High School, to develop the Roosevelt–UMC Health Academy (Academy). The purpose of the Academy is to provide youth in this underserved area with the support and training they need to obtain good jobs. Not only does the Academy teach students practical skills by placing them as volunteers in the hospital, but students are able to participate in leadership training workshops that are designed to build self-confidence and develop interpersonal skills. By participating in these seminars students learn that it takes more than technical training to succeed in life; believing in oneself is a key component to building a successful and rewarding career.

The Academy began in 1996 with preliminary meetings between representatives from University Medical Center, Roosevelt High School, and Duncan Polytechnical High School. The Fresno Unified School District agreed to seed the Academy's development with $10,000. The first group of students (freshmen) was called in to participate in these planning meetings. This idea of including the students in all aspects of program development would become a staple of this initiative; so much so that representatives from the California Department of Education remarked that they had never seen a program with such deep level of student ownership.

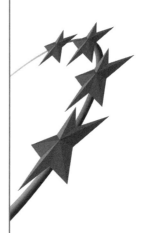

University Medical Center

Fresno, Calif.

The following year, an eager group of sophomores visited campuses of several regional academic medical centers. They listened to presentations made by representatives from various clinical departments and even viewed an autopsy.

As juniors, students participated in a hospital occupations program five days a week. The students worked in 22 departments at UMC. All students participated in special projects. They had a great time painting the helipad and participating in a paramedic toxic waste drill that had local media in attendance. They took field trips to several University of California campuses. Three students attended the National Youth Leadership Forum on Medicine at UC Berkeley and one student attended the Hispanic Medical Leadership Conference in Washington, D.C. More than 100 parents attended a year-end banquet with the students.

As this first group of seniors prepared to graduate, plans were made to further improve the program. Academy leaders continued to apply for grant funding. Ties between Roosevelt and UMC were strengthened as those students rotated through 28 departments at the medical center. Students attended a leadership seminar at nearby Wonder Valley Ranch and set up peer-mentoring groups to help each other through different areas of academic weakness. Seniors began their quest to become certified nurse anesthetists through a nurse occupations class at Duncan Polytechnical High School. Three of these students qualified for a state competition in health skills. Seven members were invited to give a presentation on the Academy model for the Tech Prep Conference at the Disneyland Hotel.

Soon after the founding members graduated, a new senior class was planning its final year. That year's group of seniors was determined to focus on academics and set timelines for college applications and scholarship/grant application filing.

Roosevelt High School has a dropout rate of 40% but only one student enrolled in the Academy that year dropped out. The graduating class had 20 students and of those, 13 completed training to become certified nursing assistants. Four students from the Academy are currently working in permanent positions at University Medical Center.

The Roosevelt–UMC Health Academy is clearly making a difference in the lives of many young people and is an important catalyst for change in this neighborhood and beyond.

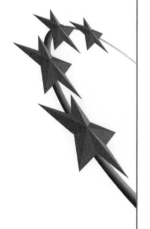

University Medical Center

Fresno, Calif.

Many believe the time to begin recruiting nurses is before they are trained. Fairview Lakes Regional Medical Center developed "Introduction to Health Care" to give high school students the opportunity to explore 12 health professions, complete a 75 hour nursing course with 20 hours of clinical experience, and earn 6 post-secondary credits. The program provides real-life learning and employment opportunities to college and vocationally bound students while satisfying future regional workforce needs.

Fairview Lakes Regional Medical Center saw an opportunity to attract more young people to health care careers when our local high school expressed interest in developing courses that would prepare students for the real world. We conducted a feasibility study of students, parents, and staff. Students said they wanted to experience what it means to be a health care worker. They also wanted to be able to explore a variety of careers before deciding on one.

Introduction to Health Care is two-term course for 11th and 12th grade students who are considering health care careers. Speakers and site visits provide students with first-hand knowledge of a dozen different health-related careers. The program is headed by our director of community outreach. Speakers include professional staff working in high-need fields such as nursing, pharmacy, diagnostics, laboratory, and surgery/anesthesia. Providers, including a dentist, a chiropractor, and a chemical dependency counselor from the renowned Hazelden Foundation, also take part. Students receive 75 hours of nursing assistant training in a fully equipped classroom and 20 hours of clinical experience at a local nursing home. They do not pay tuition while learning skills for employment as nursing students during and after high school and while they are in college. Course graduates are eligible for the state's nursing assistant registered exam and can begin working immediately as nursing assistants if they choose. A high percentage of students complete the course and 90% of the graduates say they intend to pursue health care careers.

The course has shown continuous growth and is now a popular elective in three high schools. Over a period of four years, enrollment has grown from 53 students to 120 students. Ninety-three percent of the enrollees complete the course and between 86% and 90% of the students at each campus take the nursing assistant exam. The program gives interested students direction in choosing careers in health care. As one student wrote, *"In the beginning, I was a little interested in nursing for my career but after clinicals, it made my decision clear ... I do want to become a RN."*

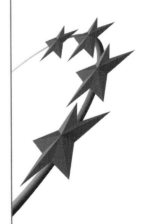

Fairview Lakes Regional Medical Center
Wyoming, Minn.

Over previous decades, many hospital-based nursing programs were abandoned because of declining enrollment and the shortage of funds to keep them running. This was particularly consequential to rural communities where nurses trained locally and remained after graduation. Feeling the detrimental effects of the loss of a vocational nursing program that had closed more than 20 years earlier, East Texas Medical Center Crockett investigated opening another program. A series of inquiries resulted in enthusiastic support from government agencies, community groups, and a local college, and the Angelina College School of Vocational Nursing at East Texas Medical Center Crockett was eventually opened. Nine of the 10 graduates in the first class accepted positions to work in the community.

The Angelina College School of Vocational Nursing at East Texas Medical Center (ETMC) Crockett came about as the result of the vision, perseverance and commitment of many people. We created a partnership that included our medical staff, the Houston County Hospital District Board, the administration and staff of ETMC Crockett, East Texas Medical Center Regional Healthcare System, local health care providers, and our community as a whole. The result of this partnership was the acceptance of the first class of students into the school in August and the opening of an education center to house that school the following spring.

For many years a hospital-based School of Vocational Nursing existed in Crockett. The school was a part of the Houston County Hospital, which bore the burden of maintaining the school financially. During the late '80s when changes in reimbursement caused many small rural hospitals to evaluate their budgetary requirements, the painful decision was made to close the school.

The impact of this closing was felt by all health care providers in our area. Members of the medical staff felt strongly that the school had been a critical component in our continuing efforts to provide the best care possible to patients. This included not only the time they spent in the hospital as inpatients but later, if they required continuing care, whether this was in a long term care facility or through a home health network.

The medical staff requested that we pursue the idea of reopening the school. Unfortunately, this was not an option. We learned that once a school has closed, it is necessary to apply to the Board of Vocational Nurse Examiners to start a program. Our initial contact with this board actually surprised us. We thought that with the excellent system of higher education that is available in our state, hospital-based schools were a thing of the past. We found that the board strongly supported hospital-based schools in rural Texas. Although the guidelines for opening a school are stringent, they assured us our objectives were achievable.

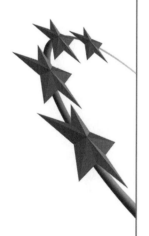

***East Texas
Medical Center***

Crockett, Texas

After months of planning and data collection we were ready for a step in the process called the pre-application interview with the board. The board evaluates the adequacy of the student population, adequacy of job openings for the graduates, and evidence of commitment to the project.

We learned that we would need to contact a nearby college that had a nursing program to be certain they would not object to our proposal. Angelina College has a very strong school of nursing that is located in Lufkin, 50 miles away. As a community college, it is truly committed to the residents of East Texas. Imagine our surprise when, in response to a letter from our administrator, we received a call from the director of health careers who expressed enthusiastic support for the idea and a desire to participate. By partnering with Angelina College, our students would gain in two ways: all of the hours they took for college credit would be transferable, and they would be eligible for financial aid that we were not able to offer as a hospital-based school.

Several meetings later, an agreement was reached between our administrator and the college president to continue with the application process for a school that would be a part of the college but physically located in Crockett. As our dream became a reality, more players joined our game. One of our questions was: Where would we hold classes?

We are currently a part of East Texas Medical Center Regional Health Care System, but the Houston County Hospital District is the taxing entity that supports the health care needs of the district. The district has a board of elected representatives that meets regularly and is active in decisions that impact the lives of constituents.

The board believed that providing funds for the construction of an education center would be a win-win situation. The quality of health care would continue to improve and the members of our community would benefit if there was an opportunity for interested students to obtain job skills close to home. Not long afterward, we broke ground for an addition to the hospital that included two classrooms, a learning lab, and a computer room.

The hospital district board was not the sole supporter of our project. The entire medical staff threw its full weight behind the program. They offered their offices as clinical sites and provided supplies as we set up the learning lab. Long term care providers entered into agreements to be clinical sites and every other health care provider we contacted came through with whatever support we needed. Local service organizations such as the Lion's Club and the Rotarians were generous with monetary gifts to set up the computer lab. We received wonderful coverage in our local newspaper so we were able to communicate to potential students the information they needed to apply. We started that part of the process with a community information session. We had prepared a meeting room at the hospital for 60 people and welcomed a

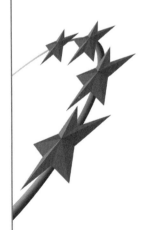

East Texas Medical Center
Crockett, Texas

standing-room-only crowd. We came to understand the line from a movie, "if you build it, they will come."

Small rural hospitals have faced many challenges over the last 20 years in the struggle to survive and provide quality care. One challenge has been recruitment and retention of professional nurses. The first class graduated in July. Of the first 10 graduates, nine sought employment within our community.

The school has provided an opportunity to meet our staffing requirements with committed individuals from our own community who probably would not have had the opportunity for this level of education without its availability locally. To date, all students sitting for the licensing exam administered by the Board of Vocational Nurse Examiners for the state of Texas have passed.

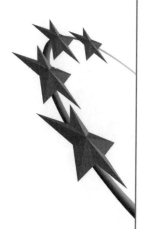

East Texas Medical Center

Crockett, Texas

Eastern Connecticut Health Network, a community-based health care system, noticed that recent nursing graduates required increasingly longer periods of orientation and preceptorship support. In response, ECHN developed an internship program for student nurses designed to allow summer interns to become a part of an acute care nursing team before they graduated. The program helps to give these young students confidence and experience so they can enter employment full-time and full-force once they finish their educations.

Eastern Connecticut Health Network's (ECHN) executives believed that if a course affiliation could be established with a local school of nursing, student interns would have an opportunity to practice complex nursing skills within the confines of the course rather than functioning strictly as nurse assistants, as is commonly the case for summer interns. The vice president for patient care services appointed a clinical instructor and a clinical nurse specialist to design and implement an internship program for student nurses.

They submitted a plan for a joint venture to the dean of the school of nursing at University of Connecticut (UConn), who enthusiastically supported the plan and subsequently got it approved by the full faculty.

The internship program is a 10-week, 32-hour a week, work-study program with two components. The first is a two-credit course offered through UConn that allows interns to gain nine hours of clinical experience a week within the student nurse role. The second component is an additional 23 hours a week when interns function as nursing assistants. Interns gain valuable in-depth experience performing complex nursing functions under the direct supervision of a nurse preceptor at ECHN. Interns are allowed to choose the clinical area of most interest to them for their summer experience.

A clinical instructor serves as coordinator for the course and collaborates with the nurse manager of each area in selecting preceptors. Nurses with many years of experience who express a willingness to serve are candidates for this preceptor role. The clinical instructor serves as a resource for preceptors and a facilitator for intern learning experiences. The student nurse role is structured so that the interns can gain experience performing nursing functions. As nursing assistants, the interns develop time management and organizational skills.

The program was opened to all nursing students who had completed their first year of clinical experience in an accredited nursing program. Information was sent to all nursing programs in Connecticut and was distributed at student nurse job fairs throughout the state. It also was publicized in ECHN's community newsletter. We reviewed applications and chose five students

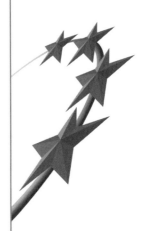

Eastern Connecticut Health Network

Manchester, Conn.

to receive training in one of four clinical areas. Two students were placed in maternity; the other three were assigned to intensive care, ambulatory services and a combination of the emergency department/general surgery.

The goals of the program were to help student nurses: 1) provide patient care and gain experience in performing clinical nursing skills under the direct supervision of a registered nurse preceptor, 2) increase their level of clinical competence and clinical judgment by relating nursing theory to practice, 3) refine communication skills through interactions with patients, families, and health team members, 4) assist patients and their families in learning about their diseases and the care needed at home, and 5) assume responsibility in seeking new learning experiences.

Interns received an hourly stipend of $12 and were reimbursed $404 for the course tuition. The resulting cost was $4,244 per student. The cost for recruiting a single new graduate is $8,000 for eight weeks of orientation, with the cost rising exponentially when longer periods of orientation are needed. The internship program for student nurses was a good investment. The program adopted a global approach aimed at developing beginning nurses whether or not they chose to begin their nursing career at ECHN.

Summer interns were asked for feedback two weeks into the program, at a mid-point and at the end, using an 11-item survey to rate their achievement of objectives and evaluate the program. Three of the five interns rated the program 4 out of 5 in every category; one rated the program 3.86 and one rated it 3.7 overall. The program met or surpassed the expectations of every intern. Participants stated they would recommend the program to other students. The one suggestion for improvement was to increase course hours to allow for more time gaining in-depth clinical experience. With the logistics having been worked out during the first year, we plan to expand the number of interns to 8 or 10 for next summer.

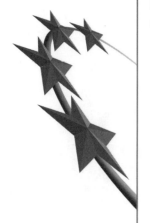

*Eastern
Connecticut
Health Network*

Manchester, Conn.

To confront nursing dissatisfaction, an alarming rate of defection by new hires, and staffing shortages, McLeod Regional Medical Center appointed a nurse liaison. This was just one of the strategies to reverse the flight of talent. McLeod improved management participation, reworked the orientation process, Increased education and scholarship opportunities, and enhanced student nurse development. As a result, turnover dropped and morale bounced.

M cLeod Regional Medical Center began a project to define specific problems related to staff turnover when we surveyed 785 nurses about their work satisfaction. Results indicated the nursing workforce was unhappy with staff support, communication, and interaction with management.

Involving staff at all levels, particularly our nursing workforce, we directed our approach. Our plan was to analyze the root causes of the staffing shortages, identify the key drivers of defection, and then implement a model for improvement based on practices that had been successful in other organizations. The team assembled for this purpose selected four best practices for implementation: 1) providing a nurse liaison for staff support, 2) involving current staff in our orientation process, 3) increasing education/scholarship opportunities, and 4) attracting students following our clinical rotations.

The nurse liaison's role is to make sure all nurses have an objective resource, in addition to their director, as a support person. The nurse liaison is also responsible for ensuring the successful integration of all new hires and reducing the number of nurses that leave within the first 18 months of employment. All new nurses are introduced to the nurse liaison during employee orientation. She conducts post-hire interviews with all new nurses at 3 and 9 months and continues to track them for 18 months.

To assist in retention efforts, the nurse liaison created a Retention Champion program. Each nursing unit has at least one staff nurse designated as a "cheerleader" who helps to welcome new employees, plan unit social events and keep the director and nurse liaison updated on any nursing concerns.

The nurse liaison has helped us create a 360-degree circle of communication for nursing issues and concerns. She reaches out to "touch the troubled nurse," by attempting to identify and resolve problems nurses may be experiencing. Many times, she serves as a sounding board, encouraging and guiding nurses to make decisions that are right for them. She visits every unit and conducts surveys, interviews, and audits relevant to retention such as job dissatisfaction, teamwork, and communication.

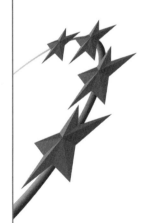

*McLeod
Regional
Medical Center*

Florence, S.C.

As a result of our retention initiatives, we retain 97% of nurses with 3-month tenure. Our retention of nurses with 9-month tenure is 90%, up from 77%. For those with 12-month tenure, our retention rate increased from 68% to 90%.

By conducting exit interviews, our nurse liaison has successfully recorded 20 turnarounds (resignations/potential transfers) this year, even after resignations were formally submitted.

We also improved our orientation process. Our goal was to decrease a new hire's sense of isolation and to build experience and confidence. The orientation process is so strong that a new graduate is prepared to work in almost any area of the hospital, including critical care units. During the first week, new nurses complete a basic hospital orientation. In the second week, new nurses report to their respective units where they are assigned a preceptor. These seasoned clinicians work with the new employees for the remaining orientation period to help them complete a skills checklist, develop individual competencies, and become acquainted with other employees.

McLeod offers all employees various education and scholarship programs in their pursuit of bachelor's, master's and specialist degrees. Many have worked their way from technician to licensed practical nurse to registered nurse to clinical nurse specialist using McLeod financial support. We also offer nursing scholarships to eligible students entering nursing school. Following graduation, the scholarship recipients apply for full-time positions and if accepted into employment, the scholarship is forgiven at a monthly prorated rate.

Our Nursing Extern program is designed to attract nursing students after their clinical rotations. We developed three nursing assistant levels and one licensed practical nurse (LPN) level that allow student nurses to enter the hospital workforce as soon as they are enrolled in nursing school. This early exposure orients them to the hospital environment, helps them in their clinical studies, prepares them to assume nursing responsibilities after graduation and shortens the orientation requirements after they join the staff. We have seen student confidence soar as hospital life becomes second nature to them. The pay is increased at each level so a new graduate is paid the full LPN rate.

McLeod has also designed a program for students that elect to take the LPN state nursing boards while continuing to pursue their RN degrees. Once students complete the LPN requirements, they are promoted to LPN Interns and work in a limited LPN capacity while completing the remainder of their coursework. These students then enter the workforce as RNs with reduced needs for orientation.

Since our program started, retention is up and vacancies are down. Our turnover rate has dropped from 15% to <1%. The 20 referenced "turnarounds" saved McLeod over $1 million. Nursing students now seek out hospital positions while in school.

The retention champions started a scrapbook project that chronicles the history of nursing at McLeod and this period in the life of our medical center certainly will be memorialized as one of positive change and significant growth.

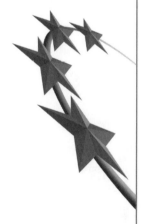

*McLeod
Regional
Medical Center*

Florence, S.C.

In some instances, even retention bonuses and flexible schedules are not sufficient to stem the tide of staff turnover. To recruit, as well as to retain, nurses and candidates for technical positions that are especially hard-to-fill, Fairview–University Medical Center used these and other methods. Despite these efforts, the medical center was not gaining the traction it needed to build a strong core of staff. A steering committee recommended hiring retention officers, streamlining the orientation process, and providing nurse mentors. As a result, turnover costs decreased, and the nursing vacancy rate declined by 42%.

Fairview–University Medical Center created a cross-functional task force to investigate methods for improving recruitment and retention of staff. By assessing past practices, clarifying employee perceptions and examining industry best practices, we identified areas on which to focus. We then identified strategies to achieve results. These included: 1) sourcing effectiveness, 2) process efficiency, 3) new hire onboarding, 4) future supply, 5) competitive pay/benefits, and 6) manager role. From those recommendations, a steering committee was assembled to implement the recommendations with these results:

Retention Officers. Two retention officers were hired to focus attention on developing the satisfaction of recently hired employees, both new graduates of training programs and experienced clinicians new to Fairview–University Medical Center. The retention officers are charged with helping new employees transition through orientation and the first 90 days of employment.

Orientation Program. A special orientation program was developed for newly hired employees, and seasoned clinicians were assigned roles to assist them in mastering required competencies and completing skill qualifications. The goal is to decrease the sense of isolation through regular contact with peers and managers.

Student Interns. Student nursing interns are partnered with staff mentors who provide additional learning support and monitor their development progress. Our student nursing intern program grew from 5 interns to 38 within a year.

Alumni Program. A human relations specialist consults with the manager when an employee leaves the employ of the medical center. If the manager would likely rehire this employee, contact is made with the former employee at regular intervals to express our interest in their satisfaction and willingness to have them return should they desire to do so.

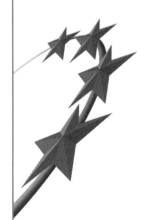

Fairview–
University
Medical Center

Minneapolis, Minn.

Recruiting Campaign. As a subset of the initiative, Fairview–University launched a 100-day recruiting campaign that yielded 169 total hires, including 123 registered nurses. It exceeded the campaign goal of 135 new hires by 34 and the RN goal of 93 nurses by 30. During the campaign, we were able to add an average of 1.6 new employees per day. Employee referral bonuses were also offered; 109 employees made referrals and 66 of those referrals were hired.

Reducing vacancies and shortening the time to fill positions have cut the high cost of turnover and have strengthed the core of our workforce. Early results indicate the positive outcomes we desired:

- 11.4% decrease in RN turnover
- 23.5% decrease in total vacancy in target areas
- 41.9% decrease in the overall RN vacancy

The steering committee continues to work with other groups of employees to assess the changing work environment, identify target initiatives (reaffirming current ones or shifting the emphasis to new ones), evaluate employee satisfaction and the cost effectiveness of our overall efforts to recruit and retain the best clinical staff in the region.

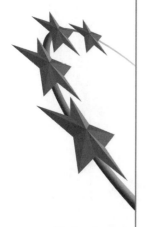

***Fairview–
University
Medical Center***

Minneapolis, Minn.

When the average time to fill a vacant position is 79 days and 59% of the nursing staff admits they have seriously considered seeking employment elsewhere, it is not difficult to understand why recruitment and retention become concurrent strategies. These statistics were what caused Riverside HealthCare to strengthen recruitment practices and improve the new hire's experience while at the same time working to enhance employee satisfaction. Riverside HealthCare used assessment tools, onboarding techniques, recognition programs and leadership development strategies to achieve results.

Riverside HealthCare was concerned about staff satisfaction and the effectiveness of our selection and orientation practices. We used interdisciplinary teams to decrease the time to hire and orient new employees and focused on ways to support new and existing employees.

The Orientation Team modified our orientation process by increasing the frequency and mapping orientation classes to job titles and departmental or unit assignments. Employees were often lost or unaware of what to expect during orientation, so on acceptance of an offer the recruiter now transfers the new hire to the Orientation Hotline. An educator fields all calls, answers questions, and explains what will be covered during orientation.

To specifically assess nursing experience, we use a commercially-available nursing assessment tool that helps us tailor department-specific orientations targeted to the experienced nurse's needs. In addition, we revised department-specific orientation checklists to develop a predictable and standardized process. Preceptors document performance feedback so new employees understand how they are progressing and what areas they need to focus on.

These onboarding methods have reduced the orientation time of new employees, and for approximately 25% of new hires, this has saved two weeks. We also created an onboarding coordinator position. This person provides support to employees from the date of their hire through the first two years. The onboarding coordinator rounds daily to inquire about how orientation is progressing and to respond to concerns. The onboarding coordinator also coordinates focus groups and surveys to follow employee satisfaction during the highest-risk turnover period of two years.

Our management team developed the "Riverside Leadership Commitment." This document outlines the behaviors employees can expect from Riverside leaders. We require leaders to develop action plans to improve employee satisfaction, and we address the results during their performance evaluations.

We began quarterly "State of Riverside" town hall meetings that are presided by our executive team to keep all employees informed on how we are performing on important metrics: financial, market share, quality, turnover, and customer and employee satisfaction.

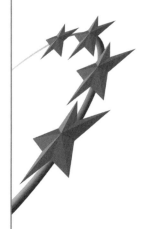

Riverside HealthCare

Kankakee, Ill.

To increase the communication of appreciation, our Employee Reward & Recognition Team proposed a plan for leaders to write personal thank you notes to deserving employees. We also began a "Thanks a Bunch!" recognition program. This unannounced, bi-monthly event allows team members to catch employees on all shifts and in all areas demonstrating our service standards. We believe what gets rewarded gets repeated.

The team also developed Pillar Awards that are distributed to individuals or departments for achievements recognized by external organizations such as CARF, JCAHO and for outstanding customer satisfaction scores. We have held several Pillar Parties over the past year and have several more planned. Our new Pillar Points employee recognition program allows managers to reward any employee on-the-spot with a $5 voucher for exceptional efforts in the areas of service and teamwork and for quality, cost saving, market share or revenue generation ideas.

We implemented HeartMath™ training to help employees manage stress. We also began training based on our new Care Partners model. Care Partners is a certified nurse assistant (CNA) staffing model in which a nurse and a CNA partner to share the same patient assignments. Our employee satisfaction survey results identify employees are now more satisfied with staffing. Patient satisfaction results indicate higher levels of satisfaction on units using the Care Partner model.

Our Service Excellence Service Recovery Team implemented a service recovery program that encourages employees to respond to complaints at the moment they learn about dissatisfaction. To date, employees have spent $2,500 on service recovery—and they feel empowered to make a difference.

Our board members, leaders, and employees are inspired by our employee satisfaction results. Among institutions in our peer group, our employee satisfaction scores are at the top. We take pride in how employee satisfaction is helping to increase patient satisfaction to the highest levels we have achieved in seven years. We believe improved employee satisfaction and retention of the right employees have contributed to our clinical and operational performance. Healthgrades.com named Riverside HealthCare as belonging to the elite top 5% in the country for positive clinical outcomes in obstetrics, open heart surgery, and orthopaedics-hip replacement.

Employee turnover is currently 9.8% and is lower than national averages. We are surveying physicians and employees to identify ways to improve teamwork and communications. And we continue to monitor our recruitment, orientation, and turnover to sustain our gains and advance our progress.

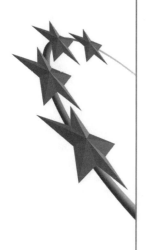

Riverside HealthCare

Kankakee, Ill.

"100 Nurses in 100 Days" is a popular marketing theme assigned to ambitious recruitment programs. Campaigns aimed at getting prospective nurses in the door have demonstrated that the bigger challenge lies in earning their loyalty so they remain. Avera McKennan Hospital & University Health Center successfully recruited 98 nurses in 100 days when it launched its campaign, but the focus of the "A Great Place to Work" program is on retention, as well as recruitment.

Employees make the best recruiters. Oftentimes, applicants come to Avera McKennan because they know or talked to someone who already works here. "A Great Place to Work" became the theme of the recruitment marketing campaign featuring a nurse relating the reasons why she enjoyed her work at Avera McKennan. Ads appeared in newspapers, billboards, nursing journals, nursing school newspapers and on television and radio.

The campaign was launched with a special event for employees. This Hollywood-style premiere featured "screenings" of the new commercials and ads to be used during the campaign. Employees received a free sweatshirt featuring the Magnet logo. This insignia for the coveted Magnet designation awarded to Avera McKennan by the American Nurses Credentialing Center serves as a reminder that Avera McKennan is known for nursing excellence.

We realized that it would take more than advertisements to bring people in the door. A registered nurse who was working on a PRN basis became the primary contact for individuals inquiring about nursing vacancies. She spoke about the benefits of employment at Avera McKennan to candidate RNs, nursing students, and individuals considering nursing as a profession. This personal touch introduced the applicants to our mission, values, and the culture that makes Avera McKennan a great place to work.

The campaign's ambitious objective was to recruit 100 nurses in 100 days. At the end of that period, we successfully recruited 98 nurses. Recruiting close to 100 nurses was quite an accomplishment, but our true measure of success will be the number of nurses who remain with the organization. The human resources and education services departments continue to enhance internship, orientation, and professional development programs for nurses and nursing students. These programs include:

Nursing Orientation. All nurses joining the Avera McKennan nursing team attend a three-day orientation session that provides a dynamic learning environment. Our objectives are to introduce new nurses to services and policies at Avera McKennan and to do this in such a way that new staff members will know they have chosen the right place to practice their professions. Following this orientation, assigned mentors continue to support each nurse with the unit-specific orientation.

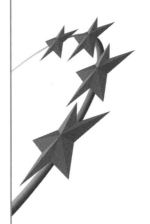

*Avera
McKennan
Hospital*

Sioux Falls, S.D.

Professional Development Program. Under the direction of a registered nurse, select nursing students who have completed all but the final two semesters of an accredited nursing program can gain direct patient care experience at Avera McKennan. Twenty-eight students have received this clinical experience and all were offered employment at the hospital.

Professional Nurse Internship Program. In this one year experiential learning program, graduate registered nurses develop competencies so they can function cooperatively in an interdisciplinary care environment. Each nurse gains clinical and administratives skills and is mentored by another nurse who has been trained to support his or her development.

Avera McKennan Resources for Careers in Health (ARCH). The ARCH program is designed to develop early affiliations with nursing students by providing tuition reimbursement and employment opportunities at Avera McKennan. Students are eligible to receive up to $2,500 per semester to pay for academic expenses and receive conditional offers of employment.

Health Career Student Program. Students may pursue part-time employment as patient care technicians within acute care, long term care and home care settings. The students gain valuable experience and opportunities to be considered for employment as registered nurses following graduation.

Employee turnover at Avera McKennan decreased 2.1% in the past year and we believe this can be attributed to the professional development opportunities we offer, the employee-friendly management we practice, and the benefits we provide. Avera McKennan's administrative council and board of trustees carefully considered employee suggestions while enhancing our benefit offerings and creating new ones. These include: 1) recreational trips for employees who reach employment milestones of 15, 20, and 25 years, 2) convenient on-site banking with the Midwest Partners Federal Credit Union, 3) day care for sick children at Avera McKennan Wee Care, which is staffed by pediatric nurses and offered at a 50% discount for employees, 4) paid time off (PTO) for new employees, with no waiting period required to use PTO, and 5) cash out of PTO accrual for non-exempt employees and exempt non-management employees at a rate of 50 cents on the dollar; to a maximum of 80 hours per calendar year with 80 hours banked.

Avera McKennan realizes the importance of a work environment that includes flexibility, competitive pay, opportunities for personal and professional growth, and options to help employees achieve life balance. It is these elements that make Avera McKennan truly a great place to work.

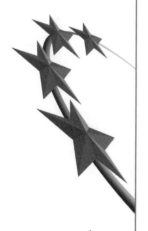

Avera McKennan Hospital

Sioux Falls, S.D.

Using contract nurses to fill episodic staffing vacancies makes good business sense. Otherwise, the cost of agency nurses to fill staffing needs can cripple the operation of a health care organization. St. Leonard experienced an alarming increase in contract labor and posted an expense of $1.4 million for agency personnel in one year. To strengthen quality of care and offset the negative financial impact, St. Leonard set out to eliminate agency use. Taking proactive steps to improve retention by offering flexible staffing, recognizing good work, and providing strong leadership, St. Leonard achieved independence on Independence Day, nine months after initiating the program.

Inconsistent recruitment techniques, the absence of retention strategies and a tight labor market particularly among health care providers in the Dayton area, contributed to excessive staff vacancy rates, which led to high agency use at St. Leonard (SL). Our turnover rate was 40% at the outset of this project. There were 69 open positions, which was equivalent to a 22% vacancy rate. Of those vacancies, 52 were nursing or nursing assistant positions. Our use of agency staff was costing up to $120,000 a month.

The problem was so serious that in some instances, agency personnel staffed entire shifts. A Recruitment and Retention (R&R) Team was called together in September to address this issue. The team put together a plan and set ambitious goals. By Independence Day, July 4th we were committed to:

- eliminate agency usage
- reduce turnover to 25%
- fill 75% of the vacancies
- reduce absenteeism by 50%

The R&R Team worked to meet the goals by offering flexible staffing, developing aggressive recruitment strategies, focusing on recognition, and encouraging nursing managers to role model and pick up shifts when necessary. Through teamwork, dedication, and hard work, we achieved stunning results nine months later:

- turnover was reduced by amost 50%
- average number of call-ins decreased from 23 to 12 per week
- vacancies dropped from 69 open positions to 11
- employee satisfaction improved by 12 percentage points

In nine months, our turnover rate went from 40% to 21% and exceeded our goal of 25%. We filled 84% of the vacancies. Finally, we achieved zero expense for agency usage by July 4th, and appropriately celebrated our freedom from this expense on Independence Day.

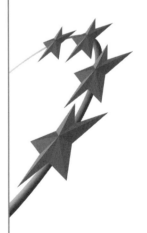

St. Leonard

Centerville, Ohio

If we had not undertaken this initiative, we project that we would have spent upward of $1.6 million. We also received intangible benefits including improved: 1) resident, family, and employee satisfaction, 2) quality of life for residents as a result of being cared for by consistent staff, 3) employee morale, and 4) reliability by holding staff accountable for the responsibilities of employment.

The key factor that made this initiative successful was the dedication by SL to make elimination of agency dependence the No. 1 priority. It became the single focus on our campus. This created teamwork to make things happen and encouraged innovative thinking "out of the box."

The key factor to ensure its continued success will be keeping it as a top priority and transitioning more of our resources to the retention side of the equation. The name has been changed to the "Agency Elimination Maintenance Program."

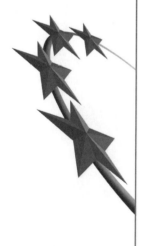

St. Leonard
Centerville, Ohio

When staff vacancies exist or employees do not show up for work, everyone suffers the consequences. This is especially true during the summer months when employees take scheduled vacations. Facing projected shortages for licensed staff and certified nurse aides, Manchester Manor Health Care Center designed a program to encourage staff to work additional shifts while nurses were recruited to fill open positions and employees took earned time off. Employees received points for each additional hour they worked during the week and double points on the weekend.

Manchester Manor Health Care Center implemented a work incentive program that rewarded employees for working additional hours by awarding them points for every extra hour they worked. This was initiated at the beginning of the summer when it was anticipated that vacations would exacerbate the staffing shortage we were working to remedy. At the end of the summer, these points were redeemed for a variety of prizes that ranged from two movie tickets to gift certificates at the local mall. The winners of the upper tiers were entered into a drawing for a cruise or a large cash prize. The program culminated with a festive party where prizes were given to the winners, and the drawing was conducted.

A winter attendance program was initiated that gave employees chances to win a fully paid trip for two to Aruba based on attendance and seniority. Additional cash drawings that recognized perfect attendance were held during the months leading up to the grand prize drawing.

The total value of the prizes was doubled during the second year and costs for each year were as follow:

- Year 1 – $16,247

- Year 2 – $39,180

- Year 3 – $40,851

- Year 4 – $19,514

Costs decreased dramatically in the fourth year because all open positions had been filled and the program was used predominantly for vacation coverage.

This successful program has been revamped each year and has been used successfully for four years. Staffing has been solid and consistent each summer since the program's inception. Our employees' demonstrations of commitment have been rewarding and rewarded.

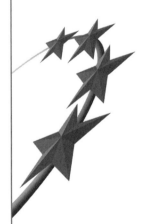

Manchester Manor Health Care Center

Manchester, Conn.

In a rehabilitation setting, the cooperative relationships formed between nurses and therapists are especially crucial for the sake of patient care. That is why managers at Walton Rehabilitation Hospital became concerned when the nursing and therapy departments appeared to be experiencing a breakdown in communication. What kind of intervention was needed to break through critical attitudes and growing resentments? The answer was found in the example of how another team worked together to make customer experiences extraordinary and memorable. The Fish! program became a catalyst for change that buoyed team spirit and improved interdepartmental relations.

Several years ago, Walton Rehabilitation Hospital experienced a grave shift in relations between nursing and therapy staff. Employee feedback revealed low morale, territorial feelings, and poor communication between the disciplines. What caused these negative undercurrents? A variety of forces were at work, including the inherent stress of a rehabilitation hospital setting and personal tensions between nursing and therapy staff. We wondered how we could deal with these realities and have a positive effect on morale and communication. That's when Walton went fishing. Borrowing principles from a renowned employee motivational program called "Fish!", we took the first steps to create a simple but effective campaign to bring the team back together.

The ideals of Fish! originated at the world-famous Pike Place Fish market in Seattle, Wash., which was transformed from a workplace of drudgery to one of excitement and fulfillment. Fish! is based on the idea that people like to work in an environment that is fun and energizing; one in which they can make a difference. We thought if we could create this kind of atmosphere in the therapy and nursing departments, teamwork would naturally follow. The four Fish! Principles are:

- Choose Your Attitude—Who do we want to be while we do our work?

- Play—Happy people treat each other well.

- Be There—Don't let distractions destroy the quality of the moment.

- Make Their Day—Make the patient's day and each other's day.

We planned to implement the program over the course of 12 weeks. Managers from nursing, therapy services, and human resources joined forces to plan the Fish! program. Rather than making Fish! a top-down program, we began with employees on the front-line. We believed the Fish! philosophy was so captivating that employees would voluntarily participate. We did not mandate participation in the activities during each of the 12 weeks. In keeping with the spirit of Fish! we wanted collaboration to come from their hearts.

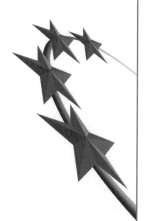

Walton Rehabilitation Hospital

Augusta, Ga.

The activities we planned were fun and engaging. One example was a "Be There" activity that we introduced the second week. Employees wrote down messages of thankfulness on fish-shaped pieces of paper and tossed them into the Sea of Gratitude. The messages were later reproduced in a booklet given to employees for Thanksgiving. Employees also contributed to a daily e-mail exchange of Fish! philosophy messages.

A Secret Pal FISH!ing Expedition paired nursing and therapy staff as secret pals. They had to figure out the pal's identity based on gifts and notes left in mailboxes. Another activity invited employees to dress up as twins with somebody outside of their immediate department.

At the launch of the Fish! program, we administered a survey to measure employee satisfaction. Nursing and therapy staff rated statements on a scale of 1 (Do Not Agree) to 5 (Strongly Agree) related to three areas: Myself, Relationships and Teams.

After the 12-week program implementation, employees took the survey again. Results showed improvement in key areas involving attitude and teamwork, both from individual and relationships points of view. Significantly, every one of the eight statements in the teams section clearly showed improvement.

In response to the statement "We generally choose a positive attitude toward each other and our work," the percentage of those choosing a 4 or 5 soared from 61% on the pre-survey to 78% on the post-survey. "I have a voice within the team and my contribution is valued" rose from 62% pre-survey to 71% post-survey. "We have clear communication as a team" increased from 47% to 55%. A similar jump occurred for "We can 'Be There' for each other and support each other as a team."

Considerable gains in therapy and nursing retention also reflect the positive effect the Fish! program had on employee morale. Walton's nursing turnover is now the lowest in the hospital's history. Nursing turnover rates steadily decreased from 7.3 % over a period of nine months, and therapy turnover went from 6.5% to 1.2%.

Patients noticed the difference too, as demonstrated by noteworthy changes in patient satisfaction. Within six months, satisfaction with nursing increased from 80.7% to 88.3%. Satisfaction scores also showed positive gains for physical, occupational, and speech therapists. Overall ratings on staff sensitivity and attitude increased 83.3% to 86% and 86.5% to 91.1%, respectively.

The success of the program was measured in other ways. The program was implemented hospital-wide after its introduction to nursing and therapy services. We could see, hear and feel a difference among the therapy and nursing staffs, as well as throughout the entire hospital.

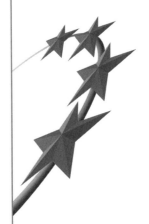

Walton
Rehabilitation
Hospital

Augusta, Ga.

We often hear and see employees using the language and behaviors evidenced in Fish! For example: Nursing wanted to do something nice for the therapy staff so they invited them to a potluck lunch in the nursing department. The therapists were astounded by the luncheon spread and overcome with gratitude. They responded with a giant thank-you card and by throwing a breakfast for the night nursing staff and lunch and dinner pizza parties for the day and evening shifts.

Nursing employees believe the Fish! program has been so successful that they are making a poster presentation to deliver at a professional meeting cleverly titled, "Nursing and Therapy: I Now Pronounce You an Interdisciplinary Team," and the poster is adorned with a picture of two kissing fish.

Patients are reaping the rewards of this marriage as the disciplines work together to accomplish rehabilitation goals.

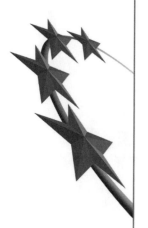

Walton Rehabilitation Hospital

Augusta, Ga.

Teamwork is multi-dimensional. It exists on a horizontal continuum as employees work together to achieve a common goal. It also exists on a vertical plane as individuals at all levels of the organization understand their interdependent roles and relationships. United Health Services Hospitals created the "Walk in My Shoes" shadowing program to bridge perceptual gaps and foster a greater sense of team spirit between management and line staff. The program contributed to a decline in employee turnover, and shadowing is now an expectation of everyone's job performance.

In the spirit of our mission to serve the people of our region, United Health Services (UHS) Hospitals has a goal to become a "Great Place to Work and a Great Place to Receive Care." Our efforts to improve patient and employee satisfaction throughout our system of two acute care hospitals and seven family care centers are addressed through a program called "The Campaign for Excellence." We assembled numerous teams to address needs identified through this initiative.

The Inpatient Satisfaction Team created a unique shadowing project called "Walk in My Shoes." The primary goal of the program was to bridge a gap; the "disconnect" that is perceived to exist between management and front-line employees in most organizations. The pilot project was initially implemented over a period of three days. Managers and unit assistants were paired together for four hour intervals, and together, they bathed, fed, listened to, and walked with patients. This exposure enabled managers to work "in the trenches" and obtain an understanding of and appreciation for the work performed by unit assistants on a daily basis.

Managers from all departments participated, not just those whose departments were routinely involved in providing direct patient care. After the program was completed, we received evaluations from the unit assistants and managers. The positive evaluations revealed the success of the project. Managers were surprised to learn how much time unit assistants spent with patients and were held "in awe" of how skillfully they executed their demanding responsibilities. Comments from managers included, "We don't pay them enough to do this job," and "I learned that people in scrubs are easily ignored because I walked by people I know who did not acknowledge me while I was dressed in scrubs." Unit assistants liked showing the managers what they do and appreciated their willingness to pitch in to do everything they could to help. Managers came away from this program with a greater understanding of the essential role a unit assistant plays in creating a positive patient experience.

With the feedback and outcomes from the pilot project, the Inpatient Satisfaction Team initiated a second phase that expanded shadowing activities to ancillary departments such as transportation, radiology, laboratory and

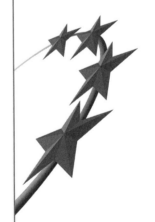

***United Health
Services Hospitals***

Johnson City, N.Y.

dietary. This exposed many managers to areas they were less familiar with. Following this phase, some adjustments to the program were made. Specific guidelines were drafted to give participants a better idea of how to make the most of the shadowing experience.

The program has been a resounding success. The participants have been enthusiastic, their evaluations have been positive, and their comments have been insightful. We also value the program in terms of its effect on employee turnover. During this past year, UHS Hospitals experienced a 7.4% decline in turnover. Although "Walk In My Shoes" was not the only initiative undertaken to improve employee retention, we know the program has contributed to employee satisfaction and appreciation.

The "Walk in My Shoes" program has been institutionalized, and it is scheduled to occur throughout the year. One other positive impact that was not anticipated is the impressions this program creates among patients. When our president walks into a room carrying a meal tray, patients are surprised and favorably impressed!

When we began the program, there was concern about the time that would be required for managers to be away from their other responsibilities and therefore, "off the job." That attitude has changed considerably because shadowing by managers of line employees is now an "on the job" responsibility. Participation in the "Walk in My Shoes" program is a performance expectation and is now addressed in managers' performance appraisals.

"Walk in My Shoes" has enhanced cross-departmental relations and communications while assuring that everyone among our staff of 3,000 gets to know and appreciate each other. The program has been a big boost to "team spirit," and that is changing the culture of our organization. As one employee said, "We're all in this together." As "The Campaign for Excellence" continues, we are mindful of the important ways this inclusive orientation contributes to everyone's job performance and satisfaction. The closer proximity of managers and employees as work is performed helps to identify areas of opportunity in performance improvement and leadership development. It also strengthens our commitment to the mission and goals of UHS Hospitals.

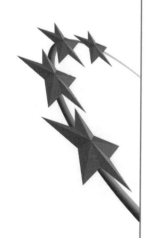

United Health Services Hospitals

Johnson City, N.Y.

A scholarship program can be a good recruitment and retention strategy and as La Posada at Park Centre discovered, it can also contribute to resident and employee satisfaction. A Resident Scholarship Committee made up of volunteer residents was formed to oversee an educational support program that funds the cost of tuition or books for employees. On-site skill training and career counseling are provided or arranged by residents. The program is funded entirely through resident donations.

We believe that La Posada's mission to serve is directly affected by our ability to recruit and retain the best employees. It is through these employees that La Posada is able to fulfill its mission to "maximize the well-being and care of the seniors we serve."

For years, La Posada residents asked how they could contribute to the development of the young people around them. La Posada's chief operating officer invited a group of residents, each selected for their background and interest in education, to form a Resident Scholarship Committee and develop ways to support employees in their educational pursuits. The scholarship program quickly expanded to include:

Summer Internship Program. La Posada recruits student interns from local area high schools and places them in areas that match their expressed interests. Interns receive a stipend from the scholarship fund. We believe this is a valuable way to introduce future potential employees to our organization and its residents.

Scholarships. The scholarship committee reviews applicants' qualifications against stated criteria and awards scholarships up to $500 each semester. Graduating employees receive $1,000 awards for tuition reimbursement.

Books/Course Fees. Employees receive up to $200 for reimbursement of educational expenses including books and/or fees for short courses taken to enhance selective skills.

Good Student Recognition Award. The committee awards recognition to employees who earn a "B" or better grade point average.

Computer Training Classes. Employees who wish to learn basic computer skills are matched with residents who are willing to teach them. An area in the building that is outfitted with a computer system is designated for this purpose. Students can take computers home to practice.

Visits to High School Guidance Counselors. The chairman of the scholarship committee and the director of human resources make presentations at high schools to explain job opportunities and the educational support program.

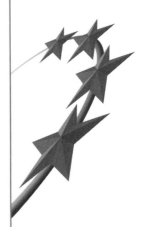

**La Posada
at Park Centre**

Green Valley, Ariz.

Career Counseling at La Posada. La Posada employees can receive career counseling that is provided by staff of a nearby community college.

Residents sponsor a fund drive to support the programs established by the Resident Scholarship Committee, which are available to 600 employees at La Posada. To be eligible for consideration, the employee must be continuously employed for six months, receive a letter of reference from an immediate supervisor, have no disciplinary actions six months before application, and show proof of enrollment and amount of tuition due.

The scholarship fund currently has approximately $50,000. In the past two years, the Resident Scholarship Committee has distributed 100 scholarships and 15 Good Student Awards, hosted four summer interns, provided computer training to six employees and career counseling for 10 employees. The total dollars spent for these activities to date is slightly more than $48,000.

This team effort between residents and management has provided many benefits, including a stronger capability to recruit and retain employees. We have begun to track the number of employees who come to La Posada and remain with us primarily because of these scholarship-type programs. We know several new employees have joined us specifically because of our scholarship offerings and at least two have stayed at La Posada despite other job offers because of the program. Faculty and administrators at the local high school and nearby community college are now very familiar with La Posada and its staffing needs. Thus, we have been able to spend less of our recruitment budget on advertising. Employee satisfaction surveys indicate a 24% increase in employees who feel that their personal growth is important to La Posada and a 14% positive shift in employee morale over the past year as this program has gained momentum.

The scholarship program embodies the spirit of mutual respect and support that exists between employees and residents, and the ingenuity and vision of the La Posada organization and its residents in meeting the challenges and needs of today's labor force.

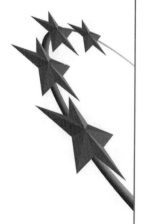

**La Posada
at Park Centre**

Green Valley, Ariz.

Employee recruitment and retention are challenges faced by all health care providers. To address these important concerns, Providence Mount St. Vincent formed the STAY Committee to develop programs that build employee recruitment, morale, and commitment. An ambitious recruitment campaign increased the number of job applicants. Scholarship programs, career ladders, and enhanced benefits contributed to retention.

Providence Mount St. Vincent (The Mount) is a senior care community that celebrates life, living, and individual capacity and employs over 500 full- and part-time staff. The Mount's STAY Committee is made up of employees from all levels and departments within the facility. Its focus is on identifying issues, challenges and rewards of working at The Mount, with the overall goal of improving employee morale and retention.

Our committee looks at everything from employee benefits to recruiting; from training to turnover rates; and from communication to career ladders. We regularly review and recommend ideas, programs, and suggestions that will encourage candidates to seek employment and existing employees to stay at the Mount.

One of The Mount's biggest challenges is recruiting professional licensed staff. We developed a direct-mail recruitment campaign and attached a gold dollar to each recruitment letter to get the recipient's attention. The text of the letter outlines the many benefits of working at The Mount and invites the reader to fill out an attached application. Response rates have been significantly better than we experienced with other campaigns.

To improve retention of resident care staff, the STAY Committee developed and implemented a Nurse Scholarship program. Through this program, all eligible employees are invited to apply for a full scholarship to a licensed nursing school. One scholarship is awarded each year. The scholarship pays full tuition toward an accredited registered nurse or licensed practical nurse program, including books and lab fees. The scholarship winner also can apply to receive up to $10,000 per quarter to cover loss of wages due to a reduced schedule while completing this program. To date, more than $20,000 in scholarship funds have been disbursed, and we recently received a $75,000 grant from our parent organization, Providence Health System, to increase the amount of scholarship funding available to employees.

Building on our success with the Nurse Scholarship program, the STAY Committee looked at the whole facility and identified five additional Career Ladder programs, including: 1) nursing assistant, 2) certified food and nutrition, 3) child care teacher, 4) recreational coordinator, and 5) certified safety and health specialist. For each career path, we developed a series of steps an employee can take to move "up the ladder" by shadowing an

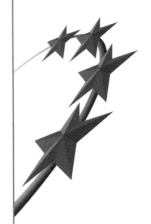

Providence Mount St. Vincent

Seattle, Wash.

employee currently in that position, volunteering within the sponsoring department, and taking training classes paid for or provided by The Mount. Thanks to the Career Ladder programs, many employees are currently on their way to assuming more responsibility and proficiency.

The Mount now offers other programs and benefits for employees:

- a loan program allows employees to finance a computer purchase interest free and make payments through payroll deductions

- an attendance incentive program focuses attention on the cost and lost efficiency caused by employee absences

- communication workshops provide training in areas such as conflict resolution, respectful communication and giving and receiving feedback

- small group meetings with the administrator of the facility have met with enthusiastic participation and have allowed an even better flow of information to the administrator

- a Diversity Committee honors and celebrates the various cultures, traditions and lifestyles of our employees who represent nearly 30 countries of origin

- regular salary surveys strive to keep all salaries at 95% of the market rate or better

Since the STAY Committee has been active, employee turnover has dropped to under 20% from a high of almost 43% a couple of years ago. The Mount achieves consistently higher ratings each year on employee satisfaction surveys. These results indicate the STAY Committee's success in improving employee satisfaction and employee retention. At the same time, The Mount has developed an excellent reputation within the local community as a great place to work, leading many employees to act as informal recruiters for the facility.

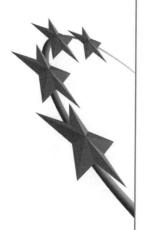

Providence Mount St. Vincent

Seattle, Wash.

Chapter 9
Community Outreach

Many citizens cannot access health care simply because they cannot get to a location where preventative and primary care are offered. St. Clare Medical Outreach travels to poor sections of Baltimore to deliver health care services to the disadvantaged in a 38 ft. medical coach owned and operated by St. Joseph Medical Center. The coach provides education, screenings, and primary care to the homeless and uninsured, as well as to the city's large, underserved Latino population. Since the coach began traveling to neighborhoods, St. Clare Medical Outreach has treated more than 5% of the city's population.

Baltimore is home to numerous excellent hospitals, but many of the city's poorer citizens suffer from inadequate preventive and acute health care. St. Joseph Medical Center, located in Baltimore County, is a 308-bed tertiary care center with an additional 26-bed transitional care unit. To best fulfill our mission of reaching the poor and underserved, St. Joseph Medical Center deemed it necessary to return to its roots in Baltimore City in an innovative fashion. If the poor were not always able to get to us, then we would go to the poor.

The Medical Center received two grants that allowed us to obtain a medical coach and partial funding to operate it. The coach is a 38 ft. "clinic on wheels," equipped with two full exam rooms, a pharmacy, and medical supplies. Services rendered on the coach include health and wellness education, immunizations, blood pressure screenings, prostate screenings, and more frequently, primary care. The coach has enhanced our ability to reach neighborhood residents in Baltimore City that would otherwise not have access to health care. Clients are seen regardless of age, race, religion, or ability to pay. Clients are uninsured and indigent. The highly-skilled and caring staff on the coach includes an internist, family nurse practitioner, health care associate, two registered nurses, a licensed social worker, and a pharmacy liaison. The coach has treated more than 30,000 citizens of Baltimore, or 5.2% of the population.

For its dramatic impact on the city, the coach has received numerous awards, including the Greater Baltimore Committee Mayor's Award for Outstanding Service to the Community of Baltimore and was a finalist in our newspaper, *The Daily Record's*, "Heroes in Healthcare" award. Our primary project collaborators include one of Baltimore's largest soup kitchens, The Franciscan Center, which services 500 clients a day, the Hispanic Apostolate, and Johns Hopkins Hospital.

With the dramatic rise in the cost of prescription medicine, the annual operating budget for the coach is nearing $400,000. A portion of the medical center's budget for the poor and underserved is committed to St. Clare Medical Outreach. Our program is also supported with generous gifts

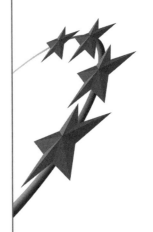

*St. Joseph
Medical Center*

Towson, Md.

from corporations, foundations, and individuals. Our economic impact in Baltimore has been substantial. Many Latinos we treat are working poor. Without health care services they are unable to work or provide for their families, creating increased social and economic problems for an already beleaguered city. With a return to health, these citizens have a positive impact as contributing members of our community.

Since beginning St. Clare Medical Outreach, we have carefully evaluated the program. We regularly examine profiles of clients served, number of clients served, and outcomes. We enthusiastically solicit feedback from collaborative partners and clients to ensure we are addressing community needs. We continuously seek ways to extend the reach of our services to meet the needs of the underserved in ways that will make a difference in their lives and in the health of our community.

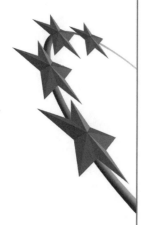

St. Joseph Medical Center
Towson, Md.

Parish Nurse programs are designed to establish partnerships between health care systems and faith communities for the purpose of empowering individuals and families to play active roles in the management of their health. The Valley Parish Nurse Program is a collaborative of Griffin Hospital and 30 churches in Derby, Conn., and surrounding areas. It is one of the largest in the country and serves approximately 35% of the community's population. The program sponsors a mobile resource center that brings educational resources and screenings to neighborhoods and community events.

Griffin Hospital is committed to offer services and programs that focus on prevention, wellness, and the integration of mind, body and spirit in the healing process. The Valley Parish Nurse Program (VPNP) enables us to help people in our community become active partners in making decisions about their care, treatment and well-being.

Started by Griffin Hospital in 1990 with five churches, the program has grown to include 30 area churches and is one of the largest programs in the country. There are now 75 Parish Nurses and over 320 additional volunteers, including church members and clergy, who serve on the health care cabinets of these individual churches. These cabinets plan individualized programs to meet the specific needs of the congregation.

Having qualified, registered nurses participate in the Parish Nurse role helps to integrate Whole Person Health into the life of the congregation. The parish nurse can assist those in need of healing and convey the parish's concerns for its members. Parish Nurses are members of the churches they serve, and they assume the following roles:

Health Educator. Parish Nurses plan and participate in health screenings, discussion groups, classes, and other events to help the congregations recognize the interrelationship of mind, body, and spirit.

Health Counselor. Parish nurses are available for personal consultations and make home, hospital, and nursing home visits.

Facilitator/Organizer. Parish nurses recruit and coordinate volunteers and support groups within the congregations.

Referral Source. Parish Nurses act as liaisons to community and religious resources and services.

Parish Nurses connect people to needed services. One of the primary objectives of the program is to connect insured, underinsured, and uninsured individuals and their families to primary care physicians. Some of the many services include helping parents and children cope with youth and teen social problems; families deal with illness, grief, and family domestic issues; and the elderly cope with the many challenges of aging.

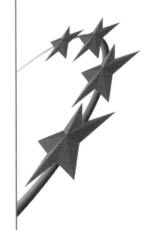

Griffin Hospital

Derby, Conn.

Parish Nurses meet regularly to share experiences, review cases, plan future programs, and participate in continuing education. Collaboration exists between Parish Nurses, doctors, clergy, and social service agencies. The program unites many individuals who play various roles in health and social services and breaks down some of the barriers that have separated faith and medicine.

The Griffin Hospital/VPN Mobile Health Resource Center (MHRC) is a 29-ft. Winnebago that reaches out to the community's underserved population. With this van, we are able to provide health education and screening services in neighborhoods and at community events and health fairs. Screening programs include hypertension, cholesterol and diabetes. The MHRC has significantly increased the visibility and awareness of the program and the number of client interactions. The focus is on preventive health services. The mobile center offers Internet access and a collection of health and lifestyle-related materials, including books, magazines, audiotapes, and videotapes, and it is equipped with televisions and VCRs. There is an area reserved for educational materials for children.

Since acquiring the MHRC, close to 21,000 screenings have been done, and more than 4,700 people have been referred to needed health and community services. Last year alone, the MHRC provided services to 8,000 residents in neighborhoods, at churches, senior centers, shopping centers, and community events by making 232 trips into the community and attending 39 community events. We sponsored 11 children's programs and one major health and safety fair. Every month, we visit 20 regularly scheduled sites and many more "as requested" sites.

In partnership with the Valley Substance Abuse Action Council (VSAAC), the VPNP procured several grants to become the Local Prevention Council for the Derby, Seymour, and Oxford communities. This Council focuses on drug, alcohol, and tobacco education directed at our youth. We received a grant to sponsor smoking cessation programs and bring the "Winston Man" to Seymour Middle School. Approximately 600 children attended this event. Parish Nurses played the role of "Samantha Skunk" and visited pre-kindergarten through grade 3 classes, teaching children the health risks of smoking and second hand smoke. The message was "Smoking Stinks, Don't Ever Start!" The Samantha the Skunk program was made possible by Griffin Hospital, VSAAC and VPNP.

Four years ago Griffin Hospital joined with Ansonia Community Action, the non-profit agency providing services to the African American community, to provide free cholesterol, diabetic, and hypertension screenings and health education for people who are 60 and older. The City of Ansonia is a designated physician shortage area. The initiative was partially funded by a grant from the South Central Connecticut Agency on Aging.

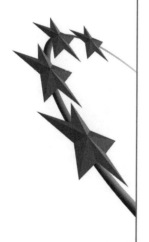

Griffin Hospital

Derby, Conn.

Griffin Hospital provides a full-time community health and Parish Nurse program coordinator, a full time MHRC coordinator, and additional staff support and resources. Hospital employees, students, community physicians, and interns provide in-kind support and staff the MHRC. Salaries, benefits and non-salary expenses are paid out of Griffin Hospital's annual budget. Grants provide additional funding and the services are free. We recently received a grant to create Health and Wellness Teams at five additional churches in the area.

The VPNP was the first in the Northeast and has served as a model for others. There are now 10 hospital-based programs in various stages of development in Connecticut. A partnership of the established programs now sponsors an annual Parish Nurse Conference attended by about 200 nurses, clergy and lay people. Other Parish Nurse programs have been established throughout New England.

Typically, Parish Nurse programs are individual, stand-alone programs. The VPNP is a unique partnership between Griffin Hospital and the participating churches. By collaborating with these faith communities, we have been able to extend the reach of our services and provide preventive care and health and wellness education and screenings to the community.

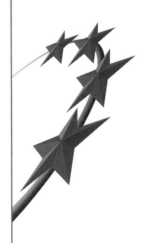

Griffin
Hospital

Derby, Conn.

Thanks largely to the crusading efforts of a nurse at Banner Thunderbird Medical Center, legislators in Arizona approved the Abandoned Newborn Infant Protection Act, allowing a parent to anonymously relinquish a newborn to the custody of a safe haven. Soon after, Banner Thunderbird installed a drop-off location near the hospital's emergency department and one night a baby was delivered to the Thunderbird Nest.

Most babies are delivered at hospitals. Some babies are delivered in emergency departments. And at 11:52 p.m. on a Tuesday, a newborn was delivered to Banner Thunderbird Medical Center's (BTMC) emergency department. That night, a courageous mother placed her newborn into a pullout drawer lined with soft blankets located east of the hospital's emergency department entrance. When the drawer was closed, a gentle alarm sounded inside the hospital, alerting the staff that Arizona's first "Safe Haven" baby had been delivered to the Thunderbird Nest.

Nearly 12 babies are abandoned each year in Arizona; half of those babies are later found dead. Thanks to the crusading efforts of Deborah Smith, an emergency department nurse, and the hospital, a precious life was saved. As the chair of the Safe Haven Coalition, Deborah pressed Arizona legislators to enact the Safe Haven law, which allows a mother to leave a baby at a designated Safe Haven depository with no questions asked and without fear of prosecution. The baby must be three-days-old or younger, not physically harmed, and the mother cannot plan to return later to claim the baby. BTMC installed a special drop-off box soon after the law was passed and it remains the only Safe Haven in the United States located at a hospital.

When Amanda arrived, the entire hospital was abuzz with delight. The name, meaning "she must be loved," was given to the baby by the nurses. Media covered the story locally and nationally, helping create more pride among the staff and community. We carried out an awareness campaign to promote the Safe Haven at BTMC. Our program saves two lives: the infant and a courageous mother. The communications program for the Safe Haven has helped area fire departments be better prepared if they receive an abandoned infant.

Although thousands of babies have been delivered at BTMC since Amanda came to us, her arrival remains one of the most memorable.

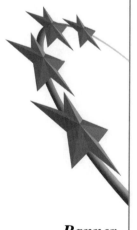

Banner Thunderbird Medical Center

Glendale, Ariz.

The Family Outreach Center extends a variety of services to help low-income, high-risk pregnant and parenting women achieve healthy lifestyles. One of the core community outreach initiatives of the center created by Community Health Partners is the Resource Mothers program. Serving as mentors to pregnant women and new mothers, Resource Mothers have helped to improve the health and well-being of hundreds of mothers and babies.

Located in the economically depressed and multicultural community of Lorain, Ohio, the Family Outreach Center helps women and their families develop their own sense of responsibility and full potential. Community Health Partners created the center and its programs to have three areas of emphasis: education, advocacy, and empowerment. Our program goals are healthier pregnancies, births, and lives. The center provides emergency assistance, bereavement support, basic literacy preparation, and advocacy training. We offer a Boot Camp for New Dads and Infant Massage. We sponsor annual School of Hope and Christmas Giving Tree programs. The Resource Mothers program, a core program that addresses the prenatal and pediatric needs of our clients, is holistically complemented by other programs that meet our clients' self-identified health, social, economic, educational, and spiritual needs.

The operating theory behind the Resource Mothers program is that the health status of both mothers and babies will improve when local women from the community serve as their teachers, advocates, and friends. Resource Mothers help pregnant and parenting women achieve healthier lifestyles and connect with health care and social services they need.

At the outset, our long term goal was to help 40 to 50 women a year. Five Resource Mothers were recruited, trained, and expected to provide home-visiting support services. We set a target of 90% of babies to be born over 5.5 pounds and 90% of babies being up-to-date on immunizations.

Within a year, the program's case load rose to 125 clients. Target results have been consistently exceeded each year. In the second year of this program, 95% of our clients' babies were over 5.5 pounds at birth and more than 97% of babies were fully immunized. Both rates exceeded county, state, and national averages for the general population.

Data is collected by the Resource Mothers and verified by the program coordinator using hospital and health department data. We maintain documents for each client and community contact (e.g., home, clinic, off-site and office visits). Clients provide ongoing evaluation of our program and have identified complementary services added to the Resource Mothers program.

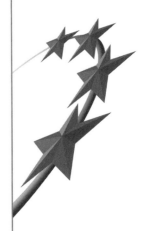

*Community
Health Partners*

Lorain, Ohio

In the first year of the program, the center's staff learned what worked and what did not. Key barriers included language (Lorain has a high percentage of Spanish-speaking residents), cultural traditions and experience, education, income/employment, transportation, housing, and telephones. Before becoming Resource Mothers, our staff members themselves often depended on public assistance. Their backgrounds mirrored those of many of their clients — single parents, lack of education and training, low income, high-risk health behaviors, and myriad other socioeconomic issues. Currently, we employ six Resource Mothers; three are African American, and three are Hispanic, bilingual in Spanish and English.

Team members are involved in periodic program assessment and planning, weekly monitoring and evaluation of our services. Team members evaluate the effectiveness of management's efforts for encouraging and using their expertise and insights through quarterly and annual surveys. Periodically, employees invite hospital executives and board members to accompany them on client home visits to low-income housing projects and homeless shelters.

The return on investment is immeasurable in terms of improved health and well-being of babies and mothers. We currently maintain a case load of 140 families in our Resource Mothers program, which enrolls a woman during her first two trimesters of pregnancy and then extends through the baby's first birthday. We also provide emergency assistance to an additional 2,000 women and their families each year.

The average cost of service for the Resource Mothers program is less than $1,500 per family. Cost savings to the hospital, per child, are calculated at $50,000 (over the first 18 years of life), taking into account that babies born at healthier weights and immunized are less likely to be chronically or acutely ill. We successfully enroll clients in eligible insurance coverage and educate them about the proper use of primary care, rather than inappropriate and expensive emergency room visits.

The success and popularity of the Family Outreach Center also helps the hospital by generating an impressive amount of free media coverage in the greater Cleveland area.

Resource Mothers receive frequent training, both formal and informal, in the areas of communication, health education, patient rights and confidentiality, advocacy, community outreach and participation. Hospital staff is trained in community outreach to help enlist schools, churches, businesses, and individuals who can assist us to serve the needs of clients. Most recently, the Family Outreach Center began offering advisory services to other health care institutions and communities interested in replicating this model. We expanded services to our secondary target market after receiving funds from the State of Ohio and local foundations.

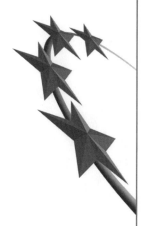

***Community
Health Partners***

Lorain, Ohio

Las Vegas, Nev., is one of the fastest growing city in the United States. Every month, over 8,000 new families arrive in the city, leaving behind their support systems of family and friends. The goal of the Family Resource Center, sponsored by University Medical Center of Southern Nevada, is to support new parents in their parenting roles and new residents by providing programs, resources, and peer support.

University Medical Center of Southern Nevada (UMCSN) received a grant from the state of Nevada to open a Family Resource Center on the campus. At that time, the center was housed in a two-room office, and offered prenatal resources and support to young mothers. In four years, the Family Resource Center has grown to include five programs serving Las Vegans along the life continuum and is now located in a beautiful, new 5,000 sq. ft. building across the street from the hospital. Among the programs:

Baby Steps. This program assists expectant mothers in accessing prenatal care, financial assistance, physician referrals, transportation, and emotional support. Another program known as "Bright Beginnings" provides education classes for expectant mothers, new parents, and siblings.

Family to Family Connection. This program has three components: 1) a New Baby Center serves as a place to meet other parents and attend classes related to child development that are taught by specialists in the field; 2) a Resource Lending Center offers tapes, videos, books and toys devoted to child development; and 3) a home visitation program that helps parents adapt to their new roles and responsibilities.

Senior Celebrations. This program celebrates adults 50 year of age and better and offers classes on health topics, screenings and activities.

Case Management. We addresses the needs of individuals by either locating or providing services that respond to issues of unemployment, hunger, homelessness, immigration, and transportation.

More than 5,000 parents, grandparents, and children access the Family Resource Center a year. The Family Resource Center receives grant funding of more than $600,000 annually from the State of Nevada and the March of Dimes. UMCSN and University of Nevada School of Medicine support the center's programs and operations. Community physicians, hospital staff, medical and nursing students, and experts in the community offer their services by teaching classes or accepting patients on a sliding or no fee scale. Church groups donate layettes, diapers, and formula. Hospital employees sponsor a baby shower each holiday season to benefit the families of the Family Resource Center. The community has affirmed its support of our center through increased participation, and we are proud of the Family Resource Center's contributions of support to the community.

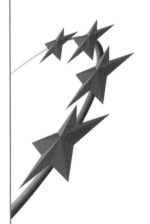

University Medical Center of Southern Nevada

Las Vegas, Nev.

Olympic Medical Center learned that obstetric patients believed they did not receive adequate information to prepare them in caring for their newborns. Approximately 60% of these new mothers are on Medicaid with limitations in receiving postpartum, lactation, and parent support services after their babies are born. New Family Services, a hospital-sponsored program aimed at providing support, education, and nursing resources to parents of infants, was conceived by Olympic to respond to these unmet needs.

Increasingly short lengths of stay for new mothers and babies can make it very difficult for Olympic Medical Center to do an adequate job of bedside education. A group of nurses got together and designed what they thought would be the ideal program for new families. Our nurses chose to expand our prenatal classes, structure home visits and establish new baby support groups to help new mothers feel more confident about the roles they were about to assume.

We successfully applied for state and federal grants to help fund the New Family Services program. Home visits are offered to all new families at the time of discharge from the hospital. The first visit consists of a postpartum assessment for the mom and a check of the baby for weight loss/gain, with discussions of any problems the family might be having. Instruction on bonding, breastfeeding, and nutrition is offered. Home safety assessments and recommendations also are provided. Additional visits are arranged as needed. Home-visiting nurses help parents cope with stresses of parenthood and inform them of other community resources. Prenatal classes have been expanded to cover basic childbirth preparation, childbirth refreshers for those who have had a baby, hypno-birthing preparation, infant safety, and CPR. There is a program called "Siblings Are Special" for the soon-to-be sisters and brothers. Parents are encouraged to join the Baby Support Groups to share experiences and learn from each other.

This program demonstrated that parents can be helped to feel more informed and more confident in caring for their newborns. Readmission of newborns is declining and breastfeeding duration is climbing, which contributes to the health of children in this community. Patient satisfaction related to the confidence of caring for newborns rose to 84% from 72% one year after the program was implemented and recently hit 99%.

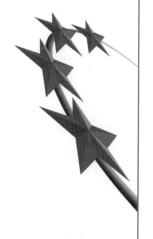

***Olympic
Medical Center***

Port Angeles, Wash.

Day and overnight summer camps are havens for young children and can help them develop valuable life skills, meet new friends and develop new interests. The University of Pittsburgh Medical Center at Braddock started the Health for Life Summer Camp to help Braddock-area youth achieve these benefits. The project began by sending 40 area youth to an overnight camp for one week. By the fifth year, the camp expanded to offer a seven-week day program and a five-day overnight camping experience serving 60 to 70 area youths per day.

The University of Pittsburgh Medical Center (UPMC) at Braddock in collaboration with the Braddock Community Partnership, the Heritage Health Foundation, Inc., and the Braddock Rotary Club, implemented the Health For Life Summer Camp project. UPMC Braddock serves as the supportive infrastructure for this partnership. The day camp, which operates from 9 a.m. to 3 p.m., is based in the UPMC Braddock Auditorium. Meals are coordinated through the Commonwealth of Pennsylvania Department of Education's Summer Feeding Program and UPMC Braddock's dietary department.

Through participation in the Health For Life Summer Camp, children engage in physical activity and exercise, learn to make healthy food choices, are exposed to arts and music education, receive computer education, and benefit from tutorial assistance in both math and reading. A formal reading program, implemented in collaboration with the University of Pittsburgh's Masters in Arts in Teaching program, pairs children, one-on-one, with graduate students. Each graduate student is responsible for designing an individual reading curriculum for the child to whom he or she is assigned. Children go swimming once a week and take weekly field trips.

Overnight camp is held in collaboration with the Kiski Prep School in Saltsburg, Pa. This camp is staffed by a camp supervisor, 18 camp counselors and two Americorps members during the day camp in order to provide continuity for the participating children. The counselors coordinate activities such as swimming, football, basketball, volleyball, tennis, aerobics and art education.

Counselors and volunteers are trained in first aid, CPR, how to deal with difficult children, and participate in a variety of teambuilding exercises. Weekly debriefing sessions for staff are facilitated by an experienced community behavioral health provider.

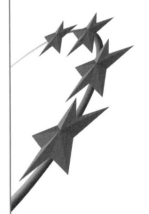

University of Pittsburgh Medical Center Braddock

Braddock, Pa.

Children participate in the Health for Life Summer Camp at no cost to families. The total cost of the most recent program was $67,564, offset by foundation grants, community donations, and corporate sponsorships; the final cost to UPMC Braddock was $18,557.

UPMC Braddock, the Braddock Community Partnership and the Communities That Care Prevention Network also sponsor an after-school program. Efforts for next summer have begun, with plans to include area camp providers and agencies in an effort to share resources and additional staff training in the areas of behavioral health. An effort of UPMC Braddock and area behavioral health providers aims to institute a parallel therapeutic camp for those children dealing with issues that prevent them from participating in the Health For Life Summer Camp.

When children and their parents were surveyed about their satisfaction with the camp project, overall satisfaction was at 4.8 out of 5.0 points. All parents reported their children came home each day either "always excited" or "almost always excited" about the day's events. Surveys of children revealed 100% liked the camping experience, 88% would return to camp and 88% would tell a friend about camp.

Health for Life Summer Camp provides a safe environment for children, keeping them off the streets and out of trouble. Their participation provides them with appropriate decision-making and effective conflict resolution skills and educates them about making healthy choices from which they will benefit for years to come.

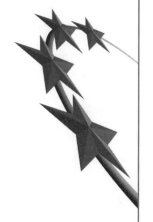

University of Pittsburgh Medical Center Braddock

Braddock, Pa.

Temple University Children's Medical Center introduced Project Access to confront barriers that prevent children from accessing health services, and to assist families in identifying a medical home. This community-based initiative is designed to improve the health status of children in the most impoverished areas of Philadelphia by creating connections, developing relationships and building bridges so families are able to use programs that will contribute to the health and futures of their children.

Located on Temple University's Health Sciences Center campus, Temple University Children's Medical Center is a 68-bed children's hospital built to improve the health status of children in the Philadelphia region. By developing outreach and education programs designed to address public health issues crucial to the community, Temple Children's aims to keep children well. With 60% of the facility dedicated to outpatient care, and programs such as primary pediatric care, asthma, endocrinology, infectious diseases, neurology, ophthalmology, cardiology, orthopaedics, podiatry and otolaryngology, Temple Children's strives to keep children healthy and out of the hospital.

Recognizing the complex issues that prevent families from accessing health care, Temple University Children's Medical Center launched an initiative called Project Access, a program that focuses on confronting and breaking down barriers to care. During the past four years, Project Access has evolved into the keystone of Temple Children's mission to improve the overall health and future of children and families in North Philadelphia.

Project Access has targeted four specific areas of need: 1) identifying and enrolling uninsured children in health insurance, 2) connecting children and families with a consistent and convenient primary care provider, 3) educating children and families about important health issues and how to use their health insurance and primary care provider, and 4) addressing the complex needs of children and families living with special health care needs.

Project Access provides an innovative way of making the health care system accessible to all by sending staff members hired from area neighborhoods into the community to provide education and support for children and families. Project Access teams visit centers of worship, schools, day care centers, public housing projects, shelters, health district offices, unemployment offices, libraries, recreation centers and wherever the needs of the community dictates. Project Access teams go into individual homes as needed and requested to meet with families. By going directly to the places where children and families pray, study, play, work and live, teams catalyze meaningful and permanent change in the health status and development of our neighborhood children.

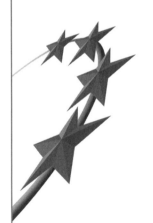

Temple University Children's Medical Center

Philadelphia, Pa.

Project Access has partnered with the community and enrolled more than 8,000 children in health insurance, identifying a medical and dental home for each child. Home visits made by indigenous workers, coupled with educational sessions, extend our reach to give personalized attention to those families who most need it. Education focuses on how to access health care services, develop a relationship with a primary care provider and use an emergency room. Utilization of health care resources is monitored until parents/caregivers appropriately use the health care system to meet the needs of their children.

With every child identified as insured or enrolled in insurance, we have estimated that this brings back approximately $150 per child to the health system for the initial visit. Additionally, should a child then return to the primary care provider or another health system for care, that child is now insured. This makes the project a financial tool to assist in improving the bottom line of all providers in our area. Project Access also alerts the primary care provider when a child is insured and thus, retroactive funds can be accessed. We work continuously to streamline the process by which we identify uninsured children and process applications.

While we continuously strive to maintain funding for this project through foundation and corporate donations, Temple Children's is committed to supporting this project with internal funding as well. Through administrative and evaluative oversight, we continuously streamline our efforts to provide the most expeditious enrollment services to insure continuity of care for children.

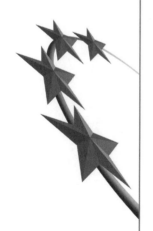

Temple University Children's Medical Center

Philadelphia, Pa.

More than 17 million people are affected by chronic asthma and this is placing enormous stresses on the health care delivery system. St. Joseph Regional Medical Center started the Asthma Awareness Clinic to provide asthma patients with tools and knowledge to empower them to combat this disease. The clinic was initiated in response to the high volume of patients using the emergency department as their primary source of asthma care. Within five months of the opening the clinic, of those patients who had attended at least one class at the clinic, 95% had not returned to the ED for asthma care.

Asthma is a chronic condition recognized as a significant health care problem in the United States. The National Institutes of Health reports 17 million Americans suffer from this condition, including 9 million children. St. Joseph Regional Medical Center's emergency department saw a 30% increase over three years in its asthmatic population. As a result, the St. Joseph Asthma Awareness Clinic was initiated based on the identified need for asthma education and monitoring following emergency treatment.

Goals of the clinic are to: 1) improve patients' functional ability and quality of life, 2) reduce asthma patients' reliance on urgent and emergency care to manage the disease, thereby reducing health care expenditures, and 3) foster a partnership between St. Joseph Regional Medical Center and the surrounding community in asthma education efforts.

The clinic provides asthma education, evaluation, monitoring, and follow-up. A multidisciplinary team includes respiratory therapists, physicians, nurses, pharmacists, nutritionists, and patient care coordinators. The asthma clinic operates five days a week. Outreach asthma education takes place in a variety of settings, including community centers, churches, schools, and childcare centers. In conjunction with Fight Asthma Milwaukee, a coalition of community agencies, we are developing and implementing initiatives to bring asthma education to the Milwaukee public school system.

Education at St. Joseph Regional Medical Center Asthma Awareness Clinic follows guidelines developed by the National Institutes of Health. Instructional topics include asthma pathophysiology, asthma triggers and avoidance, asthma attack warning signs, inhaler administration, breathing, relaxation, stress management, and appropriate utilization of medical services to treat the disease. The clinic staff provides smoking cessation counseling and facilitates the development of an asthma monitoring and treatment plan, which promotes adherence to a treatment regimen and daily monitoring of symptoms to prevent further acute attacks.

The Asthma Awareness Clinic was funded by the Clara Pfaender Foundation. The grant has been instrumental in expanding the program to allow for care and management of patients unable to afford this service. Yearly expenses to

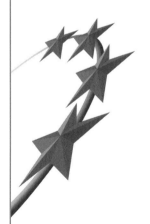

St. Joseph Regional Medical Center

Milwaukee, Wis.

operate the program are just under $75,000 and cover salaries, equipment acquisition, and supplies.

Asthma patients now have an alternative means to access vital health care services other than the ED, which translates into a significant cost reduction in providing services and caring for our asthma patient population.

Treating this chronic condition effectively requires proper understanding of medications, monitoring and preventive measures. Patients report that as a result of attending the clinic and learning preventive and treatment measures, they are sleeping through the night and experiencing increased stamina and endurance. Eighty-three percent of these individuals have decreased their use of rescue inhalers; pulmonary function has improved by 50% in defined populations, the overall satisfaction with care provided by the clinic has been 97% positive.

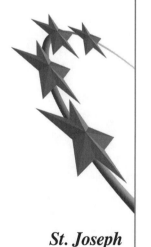

St. Joseph
Regional
Medical Center

Milwaukee, Wis.

Research confirms that 95% of older adults prefer to stay in their own homes rather than move into retirement communities. To address older adults' wide-spread preference to "age in place," Mather Lifeways opened four community cafés. Each Mather's–More Than A Café provides an inviting environment for older adults to gather for social interaction, receive nutritious meals, participate in activities, and grow as members of a vital, learning community within a neighborhood community.

Anyone entering a Mather's–More Than a Café sees immediately that it is different from other senior centers. If one overlooks the patrons' gray hair, it could be mistaken for a campus student union. Contemporary furnishings, bright colors and lighting create an inviting environment. A friendly host at the front desk extends a warm welcome to every guest who enters. Classes and activities are in progress, clusters of patrons are engaged in interesting conversations, and the aromas of food and fresh coffee fill the air.

Our menu offers a variety of well-balanced, reasonably priced, freshly prepared food that is sure to please any appetite. Customers choose meal selections from our daily breakfast and lunch specials. Favorites such as omelets, pancakes, club sandwiches, hamburgers, and salads are always available. Other entrées include homemade baked lasagna, Athenian Chicken, shrimp stir-fry, chopped steak, and all hot meals are served with bread, soup, vegetables, and dessert. Customers can dine in or carry out. The coffee and tea are always free.

Mather's–More Than a Café offers more than just fresh meals. Activities such as programs, classes, lectures, and workshops that encompass areas of well-being, engagement and basic needs are geared to help, educate, motivate and stimulate older adults who have diverse interests. Exercise classes, computer classes, art classes, cooking lessons, dance lessons, social endeavors like day trips, monthly parties and community events are planned to encourage the growth of friendly relationships and social interaction. Trained social workers, nurses and health care professionals are available weekly for individual consultations or referrals.

Each café community is set up to do more than just provide good food and quality services within the café setting. Support systems enable us to work with other organizations, senior groups and health care providers.

Three cafés are on Chicago's northwest side and one is on the southeast side of the city. All cafés are open five days a week from 8:30 a.m. to 4:30 p.m. Two sites offer limited evening and Saturday hours. Over 400 customers visit our cafés daily. They are on fixed incomes and we provide economical and nutritious meals and affordable programming. In this way we are able to offer exceptional value to our customers while being responsible stewards of our resources.

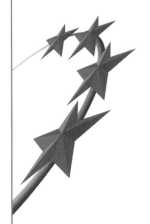

Mather Lifeways

Evanston, Ill.

As with any imaginative and innovative undertaking, we had a vision when the cafés were first conceptualized, and we continue to dream big. Our dream is to create "vital connections, extraordinary experiences, and exciting possibilities for our customers." We articulate this dream frequently because it continues to guide our programming and the relationships we develop with our customers.

Our employees understand they are the vital connections because they actively contribute to creating customer engagement. They are dedicated to making customers' experiences "extraordinary" and unique; experiences that customers will not find anywhere else. Employees contribute to creating exciting possibilities by providing opportunities for our customers to make new friends, learn new skills, try new things, or contribute to the vitality of the community in meaningful ways.

Through multiple workshops, the café teams developed "experience standards." Pins, created for each of the seven standards, are worn and changed every week. All employees are required to maintain a diary of vignettes reflecting how they have lived the dream by implementing the experience standards. A weekly electronic newsletter is sent to all staff sharing the stories from the previous week. The purpose of sharing the stories is not only to provide recognition, but also to illustrate how employees contribute to achieving the dream.

Last year, Mather Lifeway's cafés delivered extraordinary experiences to over 6,700 older adults. Results from satisfaction and quality of life surveys collected from café customers revealed that customers overwhelmingly agree that the café services/programs add enjoyment to their lives. They love the imagination and creativity that Mather's offers.

Keeping customers coming back is our opportunity. Research conducted by the Mather Institute on Aging showed that the frequency of visits to Mather's–More Than A Café impacts eight domains of quality of life for older adults. When customers visit weekly versus monthly, there is a 34% improvement in their perceived quality of life. We continue to make vital connections within our communities so we can expand our reach and help older adults remain active, independent and sustain their quality of life.

Our café model is unique and has received much attention. Community agencies and service providers from across the United States, and as far away as Japan, have toured our cafés and asked for more information. Mather Lifeways is in the process of developing a toolkit in response to the volume of inquiries and high levels of interest expressed by those who are interested in replicating our concept.

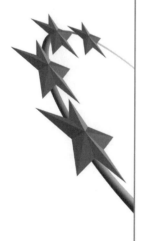

Mather Lifeways

Evanston, Ill.

One of the many ways to extend the reach of community education is through a speaker's bureau. The Covenant Healthcare Senior Health Speaker's Bureau was developed to share health and wellness expertise with the Milwaukee, Wis., community and to encourage informed wellness choices by aging adults. There is no charge for these presentations, which are given at a variety of locales including senior centers, churches, and congregate living centers.

The Covenant Healthcare Senior Health and Wellness Speaker's Bureau was developed to provide a structure for broad community outreach by the physicians, nurses, therapists, pharmacists, and other experts employed in continuing care and senior health disciplines. We began by sending worksheets to each of our facilities to inventory areas of expertise and identify staff members who would be willing to offer community presentations. We then pulled together a list of target organizations such as senior centers and groups, church groups, and senior congregate living facilities that might welcome this unique service. We mailed a brochure to these target organizations.

The response was immediate and overwhelming. It was clear that older adults were hungry for information about numerous senior health and wellness topics. Through the years, our repertoire of topics has changed and expanded, and we have added a limited number of health screenings to our offerings.

Presentations usually follow the pattern of 20 minutes of formal presentation with 30 minutes of question and answer time because we have learned that discussion and sharing are very important to audience participants. Our evaluation system allows both speakers and sponsoring organizations to evaluate every presentation. That process ensures continuous feedback, enabling us to improve future programs. Last year we served more than 2,550 people. Feedback has been very positive, and we will continue to use the feedback we receive to improve, enhance and expand our services.

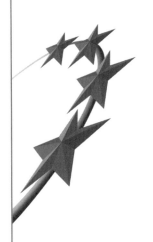

*Covenant
Healthcare*

Milwaukee, Wis.

Falls are the leading cause for hospital admissions and account for 87% of all fractures among elderly, with hip fractures being the most common. St. Joseph Regional Medical Center developed an Exercise and Fall Prevention Program to be offered at two inner city public senior citizen residences. The program focuses on building participants' muscle tone and strength, creating safer living environments, and helping seniors overcome their fears about falling. A physical therapist and a certified occupational therapist assistant carry out these groups weekly.

St. Joseph Regional Medical Center in collaboration with S.E.T. Ministry, a local community agency, developed a comprehensive Exercise and Fall Prevention Program that is offered at two public senior citizen residences in the inner city. The program focuses on stretching and strengthening the muscles of older adults and educating them about factors that contribute to falls. These include poor strength, dangerous home environments, and fears about falling.

Forty-seven percent of older adults rated falling as one of their highest concerns. Although some concern is rational, fear often limits mobility and social function, which can lead to institutional care. Through education and exercise, falls can be prevented.

During the planning stages we identified the objectives for the program to be: 1) exercise participants will increase muscle tone as measured by grip and strength assessments and reach tests, 2) educational participants will understand the need for fall prevention strategies, 3) participants will be offered home safety assessments, and 4) therapists will develop a better understanding of inner city older adults and their needs.

To gauge the benefits, participants are measured at the beginning for balance, flexibility, and strength and monthly thereafter. Therapists document problems and monitor progress accordingly. One hundred percent of participants report feeling better; fifteen percent say they experience less pain after the program.

The total cost of developing and providing this program at two public senior housing areas was $15,000. This is approximately one-fourth of the cost of treating one hip fracture. The value of this program is easily justified in dollars, but the real keys to value are in improving physical activity, reducing isolation, and contributing to the safety and quality of older adult's lives.

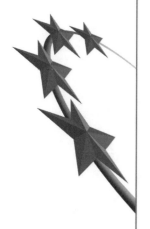

St. Joseph Regional Medical Center

Milwaukee, Wis.

Addressing gaps that exist between how older adults manage their health care, access community resources, and learn the skills they need to prevent functional declines, Terrace at St. Francis developed a Lifestyle Redesign program to help elderly patients restore previous function and learn compensatory strategies to remain independent in the community. This program empowers older adults to advocate for their needs, educates them in appropriate use of the health care system, and promotes healthy aging.

Terrace of St. Francis is a transitional, sub-acute facility located on the campus of St. Francis Hospital. We provide rehabilitation and care for patients following a hospital stay. Our Lifestyle Redesign program is based on the Well Elderly study done by University of Southern California School of Occupational Therapy, which showed that people who received occupational therapy experienced more positive gains and fewer declines than those in control groups. In occupational therapy the goal is helping people experience healthy and satisfying lives by maximizing their abilities to successfully accomplish everyday activities—activities that we term "occupations."

Our program consists of a client-centered assessment, the Canadian Occupational Performance Measure, and a personalized plan for lifestyle redesign. This plan is accomplished by a series of 12 weekly two-hour group sessions and one-to-one intervention provided by occupational therapists. Participants are asked to identify realistic goals addressing areas of concern in their daily routines such as mobility/transportation, self-care, medication management, safety, social interaction, psychological well-being, nutrition, cultural diversity, and the changes experienced in aging. Participants then share their goals and progress in the groups. Therapists sometimes give homework assignments in addition to group discussions. They follow-up with participants to ensure they are experiencing progress and meeting their objectives.

An obvious success was a participant who had the courage to use public transportation after experiencing a community outing on the bus with the group. She had been dependent on a neighbor to take her shopping and that person was not always available. After participating in our program, she felt comfortable pushing her wheelchair onto the bus and using it to transport groceries. Another participant began strengthening exercises for his arm through outpatient physical therapy so he could participate in his favorite outdoor activity and complete his driver retraining course.

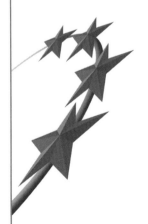

The Terrace at St. Francis staff and Covenant Rehabilitation Services leadership have supported Lifestyle Redesign by providing referrals to the program, low-cost resources, and in kind funding through use of facilities

*The Terrace
at St. Francis*
Milwaukee, Wis.

and materials. Two therapy staff worked part-time on this program. An active occupational therapy student program focused specifically on Lifestyle Redesign.

We collaborated with Community Care Organization, Milwaukee County Department of Aging, and United Community Center. A cultural exchange with the senior program at United Community Center promoted cultural diversity and eased fears of the unknown. This exchange involved Hispanic senior dance and music, and Polish culture presentations by participants. Participants in all groups took three outings using county transit buses and traveled to areas of the city not visited in many years. Outings were designed to promote community access and use of public transportation.

The program received a three-year Clara Pfaender grant from Covenant Healthcare. In the current year we will have served 80 participants through the group and 1:1 process. We hope to expand the program to a larger geographic area in Milwaukee and at the United Community Center. Collaboration with other agencies is also taking place with our involvement in the Robert Wood Johnson "Connecting Caring Communities" grant.

Covenant Healthcare has provided in kind funding by allowing therapists to use facilities, providing the services of the speakers' bureau, designing marketing materials, providing supplies, and sharing FTEs between programs. Participants occasionally contribute to costs. There have been three referrals to physical therapy, one referral to speech therapy, one physician referral, and one referral to diagnostic services. Many referrals were made to community resources: "Y" programs and health clubs, Elderlink, and Covenant's Goldencare and Memory Loss Center programs.

Future plans include serving more seniors and expanding the program to other areas of Milwaukee County in collaboration with other community agencies. In addition to referrals made by Parish Nurses, and discharges from the Terrace, screening for participants has taken place at nine Milwaukee County meal sites, and plans are being developed to begin a program at United Community Center.

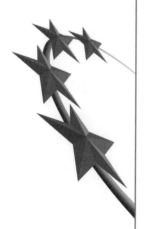

The Terrace
at St. Francis
Milwaukee, Wis.

The average age of priests is increasing and in some areas of the country, more than one-third are retired. With fewer priests to handle the workload, stress levels are high. The Catholic Healthcare Collaborative was formed by six Catholic health care systems operating in the same market to provide wellness programs for priests and seminarians. The outreach program has increased preventive care and improved health behaviors have resulted in cholesterol reduction, weight loss, and increased exercise.

Six major Catholic health care systems in southeast Wisconsin including Covenant Healthcare came together to create the Catholic Healthcare Collaborative (CHC). The impetus was to provide a wellness program for priests and seminarians in the 10-county area of the Archdiocese of Milwaukee. No individual system covered the entire geographic area served by these priests. Their average age is nearly 60 years; about one-third of the priests are retired. Priests' health insurance covers episodic care, but leaves a gap where research shows the greatest impact can be made: helping people stay healthy. Survey data demonstrated that this population mirrors that of most middle-aged males; approximately 50% have elevated cholesterol, emerging prostate problems, and too many are overweight and sedentary.

Our success with the program, provided at no cost to the participants, has been gratifying. The positive benefits of having competing health systems collaborate to present a Catholic health care presence in the community have encouraged CHC's expansion to include broader community wellness initiatives. Feedback from participants has been positive. Evaluations of educational programs have consistently resulted in more than 90% of the priests saying they were "very satisfied."

This highly collaborative program involves staff from all six systems working with Archdiocesan staff. Chief executive officers of the six Catholic systems in Southeast Wisconsin and administrators from each system serve on an oversight council; physicians from each system participate on an advisory council; registered nurse advocates from each system provide wellness counseling; health educators, ancillary providers, and other professionals provide testing and education. This collaboration among health systems in the same market is remarkable. A high degree of trust and very positive relationships have resulted from working together to improve the health and wellness of this special patient population.

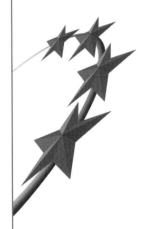

Covenant Healthcare

Milwaukee, Wis.

Young athletes are widely perceived to epitomize invulnerability but asymptomatic athletes can die suddenly while participating in sports activities. Baptist Health Care sponsors the Sports Physicals program to address the need for early detection of medical conditions that may endanger the life of high school athletes who are involved in sports. Close to 200 physicians, health care workers and volunteers donate their time and expertise to give free physicals, orthopaedic and echocardiogram screenings to young athletes.

The objective of Baptist Health Care's Sports Physicals program is to save lives. The physicals, which are offered free of charge, include a height and weight check, vision screening, blood pressure check, a general physical, an orthopaedic screening, and an echocardiogram screening. The project helps keep our high school athletes safe and provides clearance for participation in school sports.

By detecting potentially life-threatening cardiac irregularities that cannot be diagnosed through a standard physical exam, echocardiograms are particularly effective. We have carried out 645 screening echocardiograms with no abnormal findings that would preclude student participation in sports, but other cardiovascular conditions have been identified, including heart murmurs, atrial septal defects and previously undiagnosed high blood pressure. Among the orthopaedic conditions these screenings have identified are 31 noted abnormalities and/or negative exam findings, three of which resulted in surgical procedures. Other discoveries included one athlete with an enlarged spleen, one with recurring migraine headaches, two with vision abnormalities, two cases of asthma, and one student with a thyroid condition.

Since the project began four years ago, participation has grown almost 75%. The free sports physicals were provided to more than 1,250 student athletes last year. Underserved students from 13 high schools in two counties are provided health care services that many, due to economic hardship, would otherwise be unable to afford.

Coordinated by Baptist SportsCare and Baptist FirstRehab, this program is possible because of the generous assistance of physicians, health care workers, and volunteers who donate their time and expertise to ensure that young athletes are healthy. Last year, 174 people volunteered their Saturdays to provide screenings, assist with paperwork, organize the event and conduct medical exams. The Baptist Health Care Sports Physicals program provided a value of over $400,000 in free services in the latest year alone.

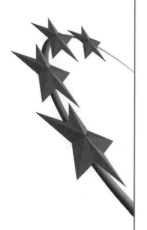

Baptist Health Care

Pensacola, Fla.

In response to regional death rates from heart disease that exceeded both state and national norms, Southcoast Hospitals Group created the Change of Heart program to promote heart-healthy lifestyles by providing resources on the prevention and treatment of heart disease. The program provides specific resources and strategies to reduce cardiac risk factors. During the first year, Change of Heart recruited 32 businesses to participate in a free screening program by offering various incentives and more than 900 people enrolled.

The Change of Heart campaign was launched by Southcoast Hospitals Group (Southcoast) in response to the high incidence of cardiac death and disease in our region. More than 43% of deaths in the South Coast region of Massachusetts were caused by heart disease or stroke, making these related conditions the leading cause of death. When compared to statewide and national averages, more South Coast residents report having risk factors for heart disease, such as being overweight, smoking, leading sedentary lifestyles, having high blood pressure and/or high cholesterol. Statistics confirmed that 39% more heart attacks occur in this geographic area than in any other part of our state.

Change of Heart grew out of the efforts of a 60-member Cardiovascular Health Task Force (CTF), which spent the better part of a year reviewing data and soliciting community input. The CTF was organized as part of Southcoast's community benefit programming, and is comprised of businesses, educators, health and social service agencies, clinicians, public health and other government officials, members of the faith community, cardiac patients, their significant others, and consumers. An open and inclusive process fostered full partnership by CTF members in the planning, implementation, and evaluation of efforts. Our intent was to enhance community resources through collaboration rather than to duplicate existing services.

Change of Heart promotes heart-healthy lifestyles and provides specific resources and strategies to reduce cardiac risk factors through two program components:

Start with One Step. A resource guide that identifies five key areas that can impact heart health—smoking, exercise, diet, stress, and family risk factors—shows consumers how to target these risk factors by making small lifestyle changes one step at a time. The guide is based on models of adult learning theory and change behavior.

HealthPass. This program helps consumers identify their personal risk factors. By completing and returning a heart-risk factor quiz, participants receive a free HealthPass wallet-sized card offering discounts on heart-healthy goods and services at more than 30 participating local businesses across the region, including restaurants, sporting goods stores, health clubs,

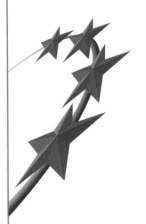

Southcoast Hospitals Group

Fall River, Mass.

and others. Participants also receive an answer sheet and explanation about heart risk factors, tip cards addressing their specific heart health issues, and periodic giveaways to promote heart health.

More than 15,000 copies of Start with One Step and the HealthPass Quiz have been distributed through various hospital sites, the Mobile Medical Van, health and human service agencies (including centers for immigrant assistance, child care centers, family service centers, and senior centers), high schools, churches, physicians' offices, participating HealthPass businesses, and public locations like Wal-Mart and Stop & Shop supermarkets. Program materials also have been translated into Spanish and Portuguese. Southcoast sponsors a toll-free Change of Heart phone line for people to call with questions about the program or to request materials. We received 347 calls for information on Change of Heart within six months of activating the service.

The task force measures the impact of this initiative with an outcomes database tool that helps us determine needs for additional programming. Healthy Hearts offers a monthly education and support group. Southcoast holds blood pressure and blood cholesterol screenings that target children, adults, and the elderly. Mended Hearts, a heart attack survivor volunteer organization, works in conjunction with our social services department to visit cardiac patients and their families in the hospital to offer support and education.

Southcoast employees from food and nutrition, care coordination, nursing, public relations, cardiac rehab, respiratory care and the mobile health van are active participants on the task force. Staff distributes materials that promote the program to patients and refer them to other programs like smoking-cessation.

Southcoast initially invested $30,000 to design and print Change of Heart materials and almost $26,000 in staff time to plan and implement the program. Strategic planning took place over 18 months. Implementation took another two years, including distribution of materials at numerous events via the mobile van at all Southcoast sites, participating task force agency sites, and participating businesses. Health care staff is trained in giving information to patients in a variety of formats.

In this project's first year of implementation, we measured success by solicitation and participation data. The project depends on the cooperation of hospital, local health and human service providers, the American Heart Association, local participating businesses, and support groups. We have recruited 32 businesses to participate in the HealthPass program by offering various discounts and freebies and we have enrolled more than 900 HealthPass participants.

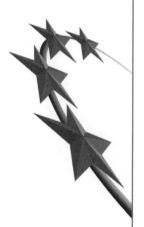

Southcoast Hospitals Group

Fall River, Mass.

More than 500,000 American women die each year of heart disease; ten times more deaths are attributed to heart disease than to breast cancer. Women's Heart Advantage is a community health campaign designed to educate Connecticut women and their physicians about heart attacks and was developed by Yale–New Haven Hospital, in collaboration with five corporate partners. Data show that the health campaign is reaching women; 48% of women presenting at the emergency department indicate they have heard or seen information disseminated through this initiative.

Cardiologists and emergency department (ED) physicians at Yale–New Haven Hospital (YNHH) recognized the need to inform, educate, and motivate women about heart disease and heart attacks. In response, we partnered with VHA, Inc., Southern New England Telephone, Bayer Pharmaceuticals, Eli Lilly, and New Haven Savings Bank to initiate Women's Heart Advantage (WHA). The program is directed by a volunteer steering committee comprised of three cardiologists, one emergency medicine physician, a cardiac nurse, and the Heart Center director. This committee works in concert with a campaign promotional committee that includes communicators from YNHH and its partner organizations.

Major program activities included: 1) developing a pin to represent the program and to be used as a tangible grassroots conversation piece; 2) creating an action card giving women specific steps they can take before, during, and after a heart attack; 3) establishing a women's heart line staffed by nurses and information specialists and an Internet Women's Heart Forum; 4) creating one 30-second and six 15-second TV ads and numerous ads for print publications; 5) developing 12 newspaper inserts for Connecticut's daily newspapers; 6) developing "Listen and LeaRN," an outreach program using a nurse and a female heart attack survivor to lecture to companies, churches, and other groups; 7) scheduling a consumer heart conference, multiple lectures, and grand round presentations; and 8) mailing WHA information to physicians in Connecticut.

Other major initiatives included sending YNHH ED and Heart Center physicians and employees a personal letter describing the campaign before launching the program. We translated WHA information into Spanish and distributed it through hairdressers and churches in low-income areas. We also developed a stop-smoking program.

In the first year, we recorded 6,254 calls to the Women's Heart Line. The number of Connecticut women recognizing that heart disease is the leading killer of women jumped from 26% to 39%; the percentage recognizing that women can experience different symptoms of a heart attack than men jumped from 49% to 62%; and the percentage discussing heart disease with

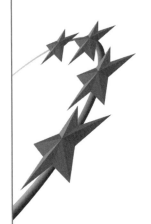

Yale–
New Haven
Hospital

New Haven, Conn.

their doctors increased from 12% to 17%. More importantly, the percentage of women reaching the emergency department in less than six hours from the onset of symptoms increased from 36% prior to the campaign to 43% seven months into the campaign, and to 51% one year after the campaign began.

Increasingly, the WHA information is reaching women; 48% of women presenting at the ED indicated they had read, heard, or seen information from the program. While hospital admissions overall increased 3%, hospital admissions for women with heart problems admitted through the ED went up 11%. The number of female heart inpatients we care for also has increased by 11%.

The $375,000 first-year budget for this program came from a variety of sources and organizations. YNHH committed $70,000; its partners contributed another $150,000. An additional $50,000 in marketing value was created by enclosing the Women's Heart Advantage message with ongoing YNHH marketing pieces. Partners provided another $105,000 in co-marketing dollars.

We learned a number of lessons. Emergency physicians and gynecologists should be included from the beginning because these two groups initially see many women with heart problems. Research serves as a catalyst for materials and program development, helps maintain and secure partners, and helps in the assessment of progress of efforts that are underway. Entry points like the Women's Heart Line and Women's Internet Forum Health Lectures are crucial to establishing two-way dialogue and relationships with consumers.

We also learned the importance of including fund development and community partners early on because they often have insights into acquiring partners and raising money. Managing the sponsoring partners requires energy, time, and sensitivity, but it is worth it – the intellectual stimulation and resources contributed by partners often fuels new program ideas.

Women's Heart Advantage is a memorable way to differentiate our organization from others as it links the skills and expertise of medicine, public health, and marketing in a needed campaign to improve the heart health of women. As the program moves into year two, we are testing other innovative approaches to continue to reach and motivate women. Heart disease is known as a "silent killer" but Yale-New Haven Hospital is turning up the volume.

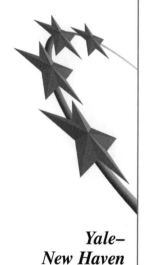

Yale–
New Haven
Hospital

New Haven, Conn.

There are more opportunities for community residents to be physically active when playgrounds, walking trails, fitness centers and other facilities are available to the public. Ten communities in Delaware County, N.Y., now have sites like these thanks to a program funded by the state and supported by Delaware Valley Hospital. The hospital partnered with school districts, churches, government, civic, and community agencies to provide support, funding, and programming to create self-sustaining opportunities for residents to be physically active on a regular basis. Mini-grants were offered to develop activity programs and/or facilities, while educational programs regarding prevention and healthy lifestyles were offered in a variety of venues.

When New York State Department of Health allocated funds to help communities set up physical activity programs and purchase equipment as a part of its "Healthy Heart Initiative," Delaware Valley Hospital assumed a leadership role in developing HeartWorks Plus. A steering committee was comprised of representatives from our hospital, Delaware County Public Health Nursing, and O'Connor Hospital. Ad hoc members from the American Heart Association and Delaware County Chamber of Commerce also participated.

We encouraged community organizations to contact us for guidance and suggestions in the development of their proposals for the mini-grants that would be awarded to fund their programs. This helped to build strong, collaborative relationships between the steering committee and community leaders, and fostered a collaborative approach to developing and tailoring each proposal to fit the needs of the community. By initiating discussions and opening channels of communication with community members from the very beginning, we all benefited from the wealth of creativity that ultimately brought programs to fruition.

This grassroots funding effort had results that were far-reaching. For example, after meeting with one community group, an existing plan for a relatively minor community picnic area project was expanded to include a playground and basketball hoop. This community had no business district or school, but now it has a place where people can gather and children can play.

This program became a catalyst for the Masonville and Sidney Center elementary schools to reinstate their open-gym nights. In another instance, the town of Andes had a teacher who lost a lot of weight and wanted to encourage her neighbors to be healthier. She worked with local entities to begin walking clubs for students and their families and arranged incentive prizes from local businesses. In Downsville, the Women's Club began with new exercise classes at a senior meal site. These became so popular that a walking trail was later developed. The Downsville Chamber of Commerce developed a map of all community resources for physical activity and is

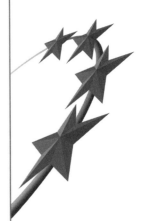

Delaware Valley Hospital
Walton, N.Y.

279

currently developing a river walk. A church member in Hancock heard of the Downsville success and applied to fund a program in her neighborhood. Roxbury School learned of Andes' success and applied to purchase a piece of equipment to begin its own community fitness center. In South Kortright, the PTO worked with the local "Rails to Trails" group and arranged a program to rent cross country skis and/or snowshoes for use along the trail in the winter. Walton's Chamber of Commerce developed a "Magic Mile" walking trail. A local bank celebrated its official opening by funding advertising, T-shirts, and free screenings to those using the path.

The steering committee also sponsored a celebration where all community participants were invited to a Healthy Heart dinner and were asked to bring an outline of their programs. This event fostered the development of relationships between community partners and stimulated sharing of ideas. By allowing latitude in the types of activities developed in each area, community participants were engaged in a creative process, took "ownership" of their ideas, and responsibility for their success.

We also purchased a "Heart Adventure Challenge Course" and made it available for schools to use when teaching elementary students about their hearts. We gave "Food Pyramid" educational tools to five schools to assist them in demonstrating good nutrition habits.

The New York State Department of Health said the program, "… has made good use of funds … and has achieved lasting results in several towns in Delaware County. The legacy of the programs and facilities will enhance the county for years to come." Ten of 19 towns in Delaware County now have new and permanent opportunities for physical activity, with the potential to impact 25,743 county residents, representing the majority (54%) of the county's total population.

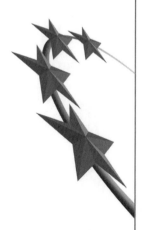

Delaware Valley Hospital

Walton, N.Y.

When business leaders in the community of Dixon, Ill., expressed a feeling of fragmentation when accessing health care for their employees because no single provider offered "one-stop-shopping" to meet their needs, Katherine Shaw Bethea Hospital responded. KSB Corporate Health Services was created to provide optimal customer service to the hospital's business partners in the area. Participating employers give high marks to the program, and some companies cite large reductions in Worker's Compensation costs as one of the benefits.

Our goal in designing KSB Corporate Health Services was to strengthen our ties with the local companies in our community. By successfully meeting their Worker's Compensation needs, Katherine Shaw Bethea (KSB) Hospital would be better positioned to meet the medical needs of their employee populations.

Initially the emergency department (ED) dedicated a full-time nurse to work within the ED creating a "fast-track" service for employees injured on the job. It was obvious immediately that the volumes would exceed these minimal resources. A physician director was recruited and an 8,000 sq. ft. clinic was developed in an office building adjacent to KSB Hospital. The hospital's board of directors provided enthusiastic vision to commit to a project of this magnitude during a difficult economic period.

More than 200 companies have now designated KSB Corporate Health Services as their exclusive provider of workers' compensation services. The clinic serves more than 7,000 patients. One full-time and three part-time physicians work with nurses, physical therapists, phlebotomy technicians, massage therapists, and office personnel to provide state-of-the-art services.

We currently supply an occupational medicine nurse to three companies and have goals of expanding to other businesses. Our wellness programs continue to see growth in numbers and types of services offered. We are beginning to investigate Web-based reporting systems that will allow properly approved individuals in our clients' human resources or safety offices to look at medical results for their employees on-line and close to real time. We will offer a Web page for KSB Corporate Health Services that includes educational information about Worker's Compensation law and as the latest theories in occupational medicine.

Construction costs for the project approached $1.5 million. After experiencing significant losses in the first few years, KSB Corporate Health Services now produces a positive bottom-line. The next five years are expected to bring continued levels of success. Customer satisfaction remains paramount in our goals and objectives.

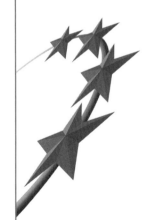

*Katherine
Shaw Bethea
Medical Center*

Dixon, Ill.

When the satisfaction of corporate customers was measured, KSB Corporate Health Services scored above national averages in 100% of the categories measured. Ninety-one percent of the responding companies were very satisfied or delighted with the quality of the services being provided. The remaining 9% were satisfied. Ninety-six percent answered "yes" when asked, "Would you use this provider rather than other occupational health providers?"

What matters is that we have been able to produce value for our customers. Borg-Warner Automotive's safety specialist claims that our services have helped reduce their total Worker's Compensation costs from $450,000 to $25,000.

Our hospital has greatly improved its relationship with the business community and KSB Corporate Health Services has played a significant role in that growth. We believe the changes we've made, and others we have yet to discover, will continue to meet and exceed the expectations of our corporate clients. We have succeeded in large part because of the patience and vision of our board of directors and administrative staff. Employee collaboration throughout the hospital also has been paramount to the success of this project.

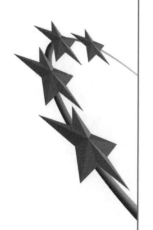

Katherine Shaw Bethea Medical Center

Dixon, Ill.

Community forums can be great venues for discussing issues and marshalling resources important to the medical and social well-being of neighborhoods adjacent to health care institutions. Children's Memorial Hospital created a Community-wide Forum as a way to bring the community together to focus on specific projects that would improve quality of life in the neighborhood. Engaging participation from more than 100 individuals, organizations, and institutions, the hospital spearheaded a project to improve the educational experience for students at the local high school. Five distinct initiatives were launched, which have since been institutionalized at the school to support at-risk students.

More than 15 years ago, Children's Memorial Hospital established a Community Relations Committee, comprised of hospital leaders, community organization presidents, local elected officials, business leaders, and community activists. This committee meets quarterly to discuss neighborhood issues including hospital facility expansions, traffic, and parking. We recently partnered with this same group of dynamic community leaders to create the Community-wide Forum, whose mission is to leverage the considerable resources of the Lincoln Park community in Chicago, Ill., to improve the quality of life in our neighborhood.

The forum was designed to bring all the members of the community together to focus on one project at a time to maximize the effect we could have on our neighborhood. A steering committee was formed to decide the first project of the forum. After a great deal of brainstorming and research, we decided to focus on improving the educational experience for students at Lincoln Park High School. The school, located blocks from the hospital, provides numerous opportunities for students who excel academically, but the school lacks the resources to provide much-needed assistance for at-risk students. While it has the highest percentage of National Merit semifinalists in the Chicago public school system, it also has a 12% drop-out rate, which is comparable to the average city-wide. The forum's steering committee decided our efforts could have the greatest effect if we focused on students who needed extra assistance.

The forum project was "community-wide" and included participation of more than 100 community leaders and volunteers representing over 30 organizations. The volunteers divided themselves into five committees, each with its own objectives. The Study Hall Committee created for the first time a well-attended after-school study hall moderated by teachers, where students have full access to books and computers for their homework and school projects. The Jobs Resources Committee, chaired by leaders of the Lincoln Park Chamber of Commerce, helped students find volunteer jobs to fulfill service learning requirements and summer jobs to prepare for adulthood. The Tutoring Committee began a Saturday tutoring program so

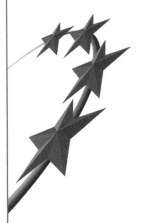

Children's Memorial Hospital

Chicago, Ill.

students could take advantage of the knowledge of our community volunteers. The Conflict Resolution Committee brought expertise of the community's social workers together to develop innovative means to teach students how to solve problems without violence, and brought motivational speakers to the school's Saturday detention sessions to help these students get back on track. The External Affairs Committee focused on improving the school's public relations, including hiring a part-time director of external affairs to help publicize the school's goals and accomplishments in the community.

These projects were extremely successful, as measured by the principal's support and the students' participation. The Chicago Board of Education agreed to fund the projects, committing $8,000 the first year and $16,000 the second year. This funding, combined with a $10,000 donation from a local community organization, ensured that the programs would remain strong even after the forum moved on to another project.

After two years of hard work at Lincoln Park High School, the forum agreed to take on a new project in Lincoln Park in order to keep the energy and talents of the group active. By this time, the school had institutionalized most of these programs and integrated them into the life of the school. The local school council unanimously voted to continue under its supervision the projects initiated by the forum.

Most programs started by the Community-wide Forum still exist at the school today. While the Chicago Board of Education has cut some funding for these programs because of mandatory budget reductions, the local school council still commits discretionary funds to ensure that these critical programs are available to students who need them.

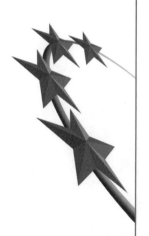

Children's Memorial Hospital

Chicago, Ill.

The Library of Congress created the Veterans History Project to collect the oral histories of America's war veterans. The Library of Congress receives the tapes for permanent storage, and participating veterans receive a copy of their tape to share with family, friends, and future generations. Erlanger Health System joined a local partnership to implement the program at a grassroots level as a community service. Select Erlanger employees are trained to conduct the taped interviews. Community response has been overwhelming with more than 400 interviews conducted and more than 1,000 calls requesting more information.

Motivated by a desire to honor our nation's war veterans for their service and collect stories of their experiences, the Library of Congress created the Veterans History Project. The project is an effort to collect and preserve audio and videotaped oral histories of America's war veterans and support staff.

Several years ago, a local partnership in Chattanooga, Tenn., was assembled to take on the Veterans History Project as a community service in the Southeast Tennessee, North Georgia, and Northeast Alabama region. This partnership includes Erlanger Health System, WRCB-TV 3 (NBC affiliate), and First Tennessee Bank. Within Erlanger Health System, the project was trusted to Erlanger HealthLink Plus. We offer health and wellness educational programs throughout the community.

The project was officially "kicked off" with a press conference on Veterans Day. War veterans, support staff, and civilians involved in the war effort are invited to participate in an interview. Appointments are made by calling 778-VETS, which connects the participant to the hospital's call center. The interview is conducted in a studio at the Erlanger facility. A copy of the tape is sent to the participant before the original is sent for permanent storage in Washington, D.C.

The expressed purpose of the project is to contribute 1,000 to 2,000 oral history tapes to the Library of Congress. The actual benefits are far more important, however. The interview itself offers an opportunity for the participant to experience Life Review, a relatively systematic reflection on one's life and personal history. As people age, it is natural for them to want to put their experiences in perspective, resolve past conflicts, grieve losses, forgive themselves and others, and feel a sense of completion. Studies have shown that individuals who share their experiences are more likely to feel increased self-esteem and be spared feelings of depression and isolation.

Another benefit is that the participant creates a recorded legacy for family and future generations. The sharing of stories allows individuals to forge connections with family and friends. These connections can enable individuals to feel alive, important, loved, cared for, and listened to. The

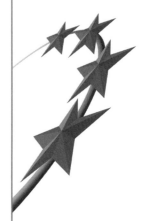

Erlanger
Health
System

Chattanooga, Tenn.

life review process is often seen as a more appealing and less threatening activity than counseling because it invites the participant to discuss the past, uncovering positive life experiences in a non-threatening environment. The studio is designed to provide this atmosphere, allowing the participants to share innermost thoughts and emotions, many for the first time in years.

Before the program began, participating Erlanger employees trained with a local representative of the Library of Congress. Interviewers also work with hospital mental health professionals for ongoing training and personal support. Emotions run high for the participant, but consideration must also be given to the interviewer who can become emotionally engaged during and following the interview.

Community response has been overwhelming. During the first ten months of the project, we conducted more than 500 interviews and received more than 1,000 calls requesting additional information. WRCB-TV receives dozens of letters and telephone calls each month from family, friends, and neighbors thanking us for the stories.

We speak for local civic organizations, veterans organizations and seniors groups to honor and acknowledge our veterans. We have presented at a number of elementary and high schools that want their students to conduct interviews with their own families. The Daughters of the American Revolution and United States Congressman Zach Wamp from Tenn., have also officially recognized us for "valuable contributions to our community."

One of our goals was to create a program for the national project that could be replicated by markets across the country. The Chattanooga project has since been replicated in Biloxi, Miss., Colorado Springs, Colo., and Manchester, N.H. It is our hope that other markets will come forward to preserve the history of the people who stepped forward when our country was in need. The knowledge that these men and women have had opportunities to formally pass on a legacy to families is gratifying, and we are proud of the role Erlanger Health System has played in the honoring these veterans.

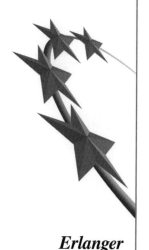

Erlanger
Health
System

Chattanooga, Tenn.

With its vision to help the Augusta, Ga., area become a preferred community for people with disabilities to live, work, and play, Walton Rehabilitation Hospital led an impressive crusade that engaged individuals, groups, and the government in ground-breaking initiatives to build transitional and independent housing. As a result, seven housing facilities with 130 fully accessible one and two bedroom units, and a five bed group home have been built.

Walton Rehabilitation Hospital may look like a typical 50-bed rehabilitation center, but our unique continuum of care extends far beyond our Augusta-based campus. When we identify a missing piece in the rehabilitation continuum, we go to work to fill it.

Approximately 10 years ago, we formally determined such a gap when we conducted a study that revealed a woeful lack of handicapped-accessible and affordable housing for individuals with disabilities. We were already painfully familiar with the housing issue, both because of our strong relationship with the disabled community and because of our difficulty finding suitable placements for clients who completed their rehabilitation and were ready to go home. Many of these individuals were transferred to nursing homes not designed to meet their needs for independence, which often caused regression of their health status and quality of life. The other option was also unacceptable; efficiency apartments that were not adequately accessible or would not accommodate live-in family members or caregivers.

Some rehabilitation providers may have been content to wait in the hope a developer would come along and build what was needed. After all, Walton did not have experience developing real estate as a community service or as a profitable enterprise. But our mission is to improve the health status and enhance the quality of life for people with physical disabilities. Yes, we serve this mission by providing superior medical rehabilitation services, but health status and quality of life extend beyond acute rehabilitation. We believe if a young disabled person must live in an elderly nursing home because he or she has no other place to go, then the rehabilitation continuum is incomplete.

Compelled by our mission, we worked to forge a unique relationship to make accessible and affordable housing a reality. By forming an alliance with the U.S. Department of Housing and Urban Development (HUD), we built the first accessible HUD homes in Georgia for people with physical disabilities.

We wrote our first grant to request funding in the early 1990s. Our employees researched and gathered information to write the application. Our therapists, managers, and other employees collaborated to develop a model for the facility. Occupational and physical therapists reviewed the architectural plans and made suggestions to increase accessibility and to add features to maximize tenants' independence. We also held focus groups to obtain input

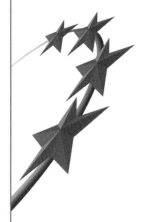

Walton Rehabilitation Hospital

Augusta, Ga.

from employees on the program's services. Political and governmental officials, leaders of disability organizations, and community organizations submitted letters of support. We also developed an Advisory Committee, consisting of community members, people with disabilities, seniors, and staff.

Our hard work paid off. In January 1996, we opened our first accessible and affordable apartments. Nearly ten years later, we are operating seven complexes, with two more underway. One of these developments will be 40 one-bedroom units for the elderly. It was a natural progression of our mission to develop apartments for the elderly population because the prevalence of disability is so high among this group.

For each proposed HUD-sponsored complex, we invest $8,000 to $10,000 in the initial stages to fund an environmental survey, legal fees, a site assessment and consultant expenses. To date, HUD has granted nearly $9 million for the Walton housing complex applications.

Walton's philosophy is that smaller units spread throughout the community are more appealing and inclusive than large complexes that are segregated centers for people with disabilities.

Each apartment is completely accessible and located on ground-floor level. Features include roll-in showers and space under counter tops, stoves, and sinks to accommodate wheelchairs. Special doorbells and smoke detectors are available for people with visual or hearing impairments.

The financial structure of the apartments allows tenants to be financially-independent as well. The complex is subsidized by HUD; therefore, rent is based on 30% of the renter's income. To qualify for an accessible apartment, the tenant must be at least 18 years old, have a physical disability such as mobility, sight, or hearing impairment which requires accessibility, and meet HUD income requirements. To qualify for an elderly apartment, the tenant must be 62 years of age or older and meet HUD income requirements. The tenant is responsible for paying individual utilities (electric, gas, phone, cable TV); management pays for water/sewer and trash removal.

Other providers look to Walton as the model for independent living programs, which is a testimonial to our success. We receive visitors from all over the country who want to tour our complexes and learn more.

Our HUD units are at 100% occupied and have lengthy waiting lists. Walton Rehabilitation Hospital continues to work developing additional complexes. This incredible demand indicates the overwhelming need for this housing program and the effectiveness of our creative approach. The greatest measurement of success for our initiative is not found in any financial figures or outcome statistics but in how these HUD-sponsored complexes have changed lives.

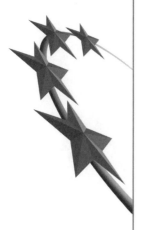

***Walton
Rehabilitation
Hospital***

Augusta, Ga.

Thank you again to all of the fine organizations featured in this book!

Kristine Peterson welcomes your suggestions and comments about this book. Please e-mail her at:

kpeterson@greystoneinteractive.com

Over 400 entries to the Sodexho Spirit of Excellence award competition are posted in the Sodexho Best Practice Showcase. This searchable database will give you the opportunity to research other excellent projects that have been submitted in previous years. Go to:

www.sodexho-bps.com

If you want to speak with individuals who can give you more information about the projects featured in this book, you can access contact and other related information about the profiles, including photographs, vendors, supplemental materials, and updates at:

www.spirit-excellence.com

Substantial discounts on bulk quantities of this book are available upon request. For rates and ordering information, please contact:

info@candentpress.com

APPENDIX

Page	Sponsor	Location	Profile Title
3	Advocate Health Care	Oak Brook, Ill.	Living Our Values
197	Banner Thunderbird Medical Center	Glendale, Ariz.	60 Minutes Builds Communication
256	Banner Thunderbird Medical Center	Glendale, Ariz.	Creating a Safe Haven
199	Baptist Health Care	Pensacola, Fla.	A Daily Dose of Continuous Learning
274	Baptist Health Care	Pensacola, Fla.	Sports Physicals Program
203	Bayhealth Medical Center	Dover, Del.	You've Been Caught on the Spot
39	Beaumont Hospital–Troy	Troy, Mich.	Shhh! Obstetrics Unit Listens to Customers
71	Brenner Children's Hospital	Winston–Salem, N.C.	Supporting Hispanic Patients and Families
85	Brenner Children's Hospital	Winston–Salem, N.C.	Bereavement Support Because We Care
185	Bristol Hospital	Bristol, Conn.	Staying Close to Customers
153	Cape Canaveral Hospital	Coco Beach, Fla.	Delivering Extraordinary Emergency Service
53	Cape Fear Valley Health System	Fayetteville, N.C.	Cancer Center Comprehensive Care
81	Capital Health District Authority	Halifax, Nova Scotia	High Tech–High Touch Critical Care
69	Carle Foundation Hospital	Urbana, Ill.	Extending Hospitality to Guests
61	Carondelet St. Joseph's Hospital	Tucson, Ariz.	PAWS for Healthy Rehabilitation
139	Carondelet St. Joseph's Hospital	Tucson, Ariz.	Ruby Slippers Reduce Slips
141	Carondelet St. Joseph's Hospital	Tucson, Ariz.	The Road to Safe Surgery
218	Carondelet St. Joseph's Hospital	Tucson, Ariz.	Walk-a-Mile With a Nurse
283	Children's Memorial Hospital	Chicago, Ill.	Community Forum
59	Clara Maass Medical Center	Belleville, N.J.	Taking Pride in Environmental Services
82	Clara Maass Medical Center	Belleville, N.J.	Revitalizing Pastoral Care
34	Columbia Memorial Hospital	Hudson, N.Y.	Focusing on Family-Centered Care
74	Columbia Memorial Hospital	Hudson, N.Y.	Preparing KIDZ for Surgery
143	Columbia Memorial Hospital	Hudson, N.Y.	Transfusion-Free Medicine & Surgery
147	Columbus Regional Hospital	Columbus, Ind.	Improving Women's Breast Health Services
257	Community Health Partners	Lorain, Ohio	Resource Mothers Program
41	Concord Hospital	Concord, N.H.	Orthopedics–Psst! ... Have You Heard?
15	Conemaugh Memorial Medical Center	Johnstown, Pa.	Becoming the Gold Standard
169	Conemaugh Memorial Medical Center	Johnstown, Pa.	Introducing Crossroads Café
121	Covenant Healthcare	Milwaukee, Wis.	Preventing Medication Errors
269	Covenant Healthcare	Milwaukee, Wis.	Speaking Out for Seniors
273	Covenant Healthcare	Milwaukee, Wis.	Wellness Program for Priests
179	Daniel Freeman Memorial Hospital	Inglewood, Calif.	Comfort Care for the Terminally Ill
90	Daughters of Israel	West Orange, N.J.	Spirituality Programs Provide Solace
111	Daughters of Israel	West Orange, N.J.	Structuring Quality Improvement
49	Delaware Valley Hospital	Walton, N.Y.	Med/Surg Unit Campaigns for Excellence
279	Delaware Valley Hospital	Walton, N.Y.	HeartWorks Plus
187	Denver Health	Denver, Colo.	Mystery Shoppers Reveal Insights
191	Veterans Affairs New Jersey Health Care System	East Orange, N.J.	Improving Customer Service Knowledge
204	Veterans Affairs New Jersey Health Care System	East Orange, N.J.	Oak Leaf Awards Honor Heroes
6	DuBois Regional Medical Center	DuBois, Pa.	Creating a Service Culture
161	Duncan Regional Hospital	Duncan, Okla.	Discovering an Elegant Solution in the ED
224	East Texas Medical Center Crockett	Crockett, Texas	Revitalizing Nursing Education
227	Eastern Connecticut Health Network	Manchester, Conn.	Summer Internship Program

Page	Sponsor	Location	Profile Title
102	Eger Health Care and Rehabilitation Center	Staten Island, N.Y.	Adjusting to the Speed of Change
285	Erlanger Health System	Chattanooga, Tenn.	Veterans History Project
223	Fairview Lakes Regional Medical Center	Wyoming, Minn.	Introduction to Health Care
47	Fairview–University Medical Center	Minneapolis, Minn.	Med/Surg Unit Engages Employees
231	Fairview–University Medical Center	Minneapolis, Minn.	Recruiting and Retaining the Best
140	Florida Hospital Celebration Health	Celebration, Fla.	Surgical Learning Institute
93	Friendly Acres Retirement Community	Newton, Kan.	Stimulating Relaxation through Snoezelen
117	Froedtert Hospital	Milwaukee, Wis.	Six Sigma Improves Patient Safety
174	Garden Grove Hospital	Garden Grove, Calif.	Nourishing Patients with Special Needs
193	Geisinger Health System	Danville, Pa.	Physicians Practice Customer Service
115	Gibson General Hospital	Trenton, Tenn.	Quality Improvement in Rural Health
106	Glencroft Care Center	Glendale, Ariz.	Nourishing Care in Advanced Dementia
27	Griffin Hospital	Derby, Conn.	Embracing the Planetree Philosophy
253	Griffin Hospital	Derby, Conn.	Valley Parish Nurse Program
205	Guthrie Health	Sayre, Pa.	Leadership As a Business Strategy
45	Hackensack University Medical Center	Hackensack, N.J.	Making a Difference in Pediatric Oncology
75	Hackensack University Medical Center	Hackensack, N.J.	Shoppe Provides Personalized Service
201	Hackensack University Medical Center	Hackensack, N.J.	5 Star Care Recognition Program
215	Hackensack University Medical Center	Hackensack, N.J.	Achieving Success Over Stress
171	Hamot Medical Center	Erie, Pa.	Room Service at Your Request
77	Harbor–UCLA Medical Center	Torrance, Calif.	Innovations in Healing–Using the Arts
51	Highsmith–Rainey Memorial Hospital	Fayetteville, N.C.	Surgery/GI Lab Improves Communication
17	Huron–Valley Sinai Hospital	Commerce, Mich.	Winning Team Spirit
23	Ideal Senior Living Center	Endicott, N.Y.	Rolling Out the Red Carpet
89	Imperial Point Medical Center	Fort Lauderdale, Fla.	Reuniting and Celebrating Champions
108	Jupiter Medical Center Pavilion	Jupiter, Fla.	First Impressions Form Foundations
281	Katherine Shaw Bethea Medical Center	Dixon, Ill.	Corporate Health Services
107	La Posada at Park Centre	Green Valley, Ariz.	Settling in at La Posada
245	La Posada at Park Centre	Green Valley, Ariz.	Resident Scholarship Committee
73	La Rabida Children's Hospital	Chicago, Ill.	Giving the Gift of Learning
31	Lancaster General Women & Babies Hospital	Lancaster, Pa.	Designing Health Care for Women
157	Lankenau Hospital	Lankenau, Pa.	Revitalizing Emergency Medicine
167	Lindsborg Community Hospital	Lindsborg, Kan.	Healthy Fast Food to Go
99	Long Island State Veterans Home	Stony Brook, N.Y.	Chef's Club Engages Veterans
123	Loyola University Medical Center	Maywood, Ill.	Computerized Physician Order Entry
239	Manchester Manor Health Care Center	Manchester, Conn.	Commitment Pays!
267	Mather Lifeways	Evanston, Ill.	Mather's–More Than A Café
177	Mayo Clinic in Scottsdale	Scottsdale, Ariz.	Easing the Pain of Billing System Conversion
235	McKennan Hospital & University Health Center	Sioux Falls, S.D.	A Great Place to Work Campaign
65	McLeod Regional Medical Center	Florence, S.C.	Giving Patients a LIFT
229	McLeod Regional Medical Center	Florence, S.C.	Reversing the Flight of Talent
189	Memorial Hospital of South Bend	South Bend, Ind.	Measuring Internal Customer Satisfaction
79	Mountain States Health Alliance	Johnson City, Tenn.	Stories for the Soul
80	Mountain States Health Alliance	Johnson City, Tenn.	Advocates for Families

For contact information, please go to: www.spirit-excellence.com

APPENDIX

Page	Sponsor	Location	Profile Title
166	Mountain States Health Alliance	Johnson City, Tenn.	Transporting Patients Safely by Air
217	NCH Healthcare System	Naples, Fla.	Mastering Fluency in English
104	Neshaminy Manor	Warrington, Pa.	Dining at New York Deli
30	North Shore Birth Center	Beverly, Mass.	Giving Childbirth Back to Women
150	Northwestern Memorial Hospital	Chicago, Ill.	The Best Possible Outpatient Experience
113	Olympic Medical Center	Port Angeles, Wash.	Forming a Medical Quality Institute
260	Olympic Medical Center	Port Angeles, Wash.	New Family Services
129	OSF Saint James–John W. Albrecht Medical Center	Pontiac, Ill.	Pain Smarts!
126	OSU & Harding Behavioral Healthcare and Medicine	Columbus, Ohio	Pain Management in Behavioral Health
9	Parkview North Hospital	Fort Wayne, Ind.	Setting Service Excellence Goals
155	Parma Community General Hospital	Parma, Ohio	Cranking Up the HEAT
67	Phoebe Putney Memorial Hospital	Albany, Ga.	Going the Extra Mile
87	PinnacleHealth System	Harrisburg, Pa.	Hope and Healing After Perinatal Loss
127	PinnacleHealth System	Harrisburg, Pa.	Pain Management Committee
133	PinnacleHealth System	Harrisburg, Pa.	Outpatient Heart Failure Program
213	PinnacleHealth System	Harrisburg, Pa.	Reinforcing the Value of Diversity
163	Prince William Hospital	Manassas, Va.	A Special ED Experience for Children
19	Providence Centralia Hospital	Centralia, Wash.	Shaping Service Success
105	Providence Mount St. Vincent	Seattle, Wash.	Themes Enhance Meal Service
212	Providence Mount St. Vincent	Seattle, Wash.	Building Cultural Awareness
247	Providence Mount St. Vincent	Seattle, Wash.	STAY Committee Improves Retention
233	Riverside HealthCare	Kankakee, Ill.	Improving Recruitment and Retention
159	Robert Wood Johnson Hospital at Hamilton	Hamilton, N.J.	Driving Forces of Change
101	Rockwood Retirement Community	Spokane, Wash.	Gourmet Chef on Wheels Delivers
131	Rome Memorial Hospital	Rome, N.Y.	C-Section Rate Reduction
138	Sharp Grossmont Hospital	La Mesa, Calif.	Preventing Patients from Falling
195	Sharp Grossmont Hospital	La Mesa, Calif.	Key Words and Actions Enhance Service
209	Sharp HealthCare Home Care Agency	San Diego, Calif.	Celebrate and Rejoice in Diversity
83	Sharp HospiceCare	San Diego, Calif.	Holding on to Memory Bears
275	Southcoast Hospitals Group	Fall River, Mass.	Change of Heart
135	Spartanburg Hospital for Restorative Care	Spartanburg, S.C.	Screening for Infections
78	St. Bernardine Medical Center	San Bernardino, Calif.	Music Ministry Program
84	St. Francis Hospice	Honolulu, Hawaii	Walk the Mall Grief Support
181	St. John's Regional Medical Center	Joplin, Mo.	Palliative Care and Compassion
251	St. Joseph Medical Center	Towson, Md.	Coach Delivers Medical Outreach
265	St. Joseph Regional Medical Center	Milwaukee, Wis.	Asthma Awareness Clinic
270	St. Joseph Regional Medical Center	Milwaukee, Wis.	Stay On Your Feet, Seniors
137	St. Joseph's Hospital	Elmira, N.Y.	Common Canister Protocol
237	St. Leonard	Centerville, Ohio	Independence from Agency Staffing
119	St. Mary Medical Center	Hobart, Ind.	Special Precautions Medication Process
263	Temple University Children's Medical Center	Philadelphia, Pa.	Reaching Out to Children
173	The Nebraska Medical Center	Omaha, Neb.	Meal Service 'Made to Order'
175	The Queen's Medical Center	Honolulu, Hawaii	Outsourcing Food and Nutritional Services
43	The St. Luke Hospital West	Florence, Ky.	Transitional Care Unit Renews Commitment

For contact information, please go to: www.spirit-excellence.com

Page	Sponsor	Location	Profile Title
271	The Terrace at St. Francis	Milwaukee, Wis.	Lifestyle Redesign Program
57	The Toledo Hospital	Toledo, Ohio	Building Performance and Morale in Dietary
12	Thomas Hospital	Fairhope, Ala.	Earning Service & Financial Success
55	UC Irvine Medical Center	Orange, Calif.	Improving Ambulatory Care Performance
243	United Health Services Hospitals	Johnson City, N.Y.	"Walk In My Shoes" Shadowing Project
95	United Retirement Center	Brookings, S.D.	Alleviating Loneliness – Project ALIVE!
221	University Medical Center	Fresno, Calif.	Roosevelt–UMC Academy
259	University Medical Center of Southern Nevada	Las Vegas, Nev.	Family Resource Center
207	University of Kentucky Hospital	Lexington, Ky.	Mentoring Tomorrow's Leaders
261	University of Pittsburgh Medical Center Braddock	Braddock, Pa.	Health for Life Summer Camp
176	Vernon Manor	Vernon, Conn.	Creating an Inventory Control System
214	Wake Forest University Baptist Medical	Winston–Salem, N.C.	Healthy Incentives for Employees
240	Walton Rehabilitation Hospital	Augusta, Ga.	The FISH! Experience
287	Walton Rehabilitation Hospital	Augusta, Ga.	Home Sweet Home
103	Westchester Care Center	Tempe, Ariz.	Creating the Dining Experience
165	White County Medical Center	Searcy, Ark.	Moving on the ED Fast Track
21	Whitman Hospital and Medical Center	Colfax, Wash.	Showing We Care
97	Windy Hill Village of the Presbyterian Homes	Philipsburg, Pa.	Safety Without Restraint
25	Yakima Valley Memorial Hospital	Yakima, Wash.	Transforming Garden Village
277	Yale–New Haven Hospital	New Haven, Conn.	Heart Healthy Women

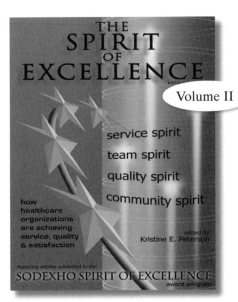

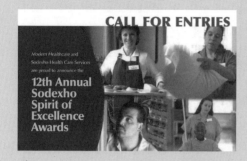
294